KU-680-960

THEORY AND PRACTICE OF HIV COUNSELLING

A Systemic Approach

ROBERT BOR

RIVA MILLER

AND

ELEANOR GOLDMAN

CASSELL

Cassell
Villiers House, 41/47 Strand, London WC2N 5JE

© Robert Bor, Riva Miller and Eleanor Goldman 1992

All rights reserved. No part of this publication may be reproduced
or transmitted in any form or by any means, electronic or
mechanical including photocopying, recording or any information
storage or retrieval system, without prior permission in writing
from the publishers.

First published 1992
Reprinted with corrections 1993

British Library Cataloguing-in-Publication Data
A catalogue record for this book is available from the British
Library.

ISBN 0–304–32602–X (hardback)
0–304–32580–5 (paperback)

Typeset by Litho Link Ltd, Welshpool, Powys, Wales
Printed and bound in Great Britain by
Dotesios, Trowbridge, Wilts.

0127272

P705
1899
HRM
(Bor)

Theory and Practice of
HIV Counselling

HAROLD BRIDGES LIBRARY
S. MARTIN'S COLLEGE
LANCASTER

Books are to be returned on or before
the last date below.

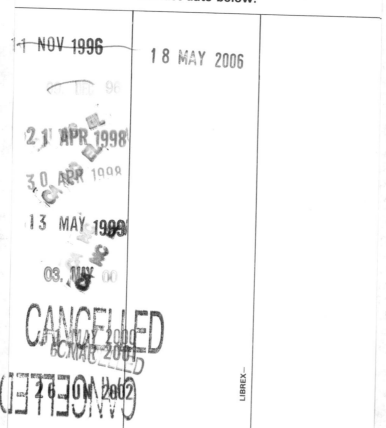

1 1 NOV 1996

18 MAY 2006

21 APR 1998

30 APR 1998

13 MAY 1999

03. MAY 00

CANCELLED

06 MAR 2001

CANCELLED

26 NOV 2002

LIBREX—

030432580

Available in the Cassell Education series:

P. Ainley: *Young People Leaving Home*

P. Ainley and M. Corney: *Training for the Future: The Rise and Fall of the Manpower Services Commission*

G. Antonouris and J. Wilson: *Equal Opportunities in Schools: New Dimensions in Topic Work*

L. Bash and D. Coulby: *The Education Reform Act: Competition and Control*

D. E. Bland: *Managing Higher Education*

M. Booth, J. Furlong and M. Wilkin: *Partnership in Initial Teacher Training*

M. Bottery: *The Morality of the School*

G. Claxton: *Being a Teacher: A Positive Approach to Change and Stress*

G. Claxton: *Teaching to Learn: A Direction for Education*

D. Coulby and L. Bash: *Contradiction and Conflict: The 1988 Education Act in Action*

D. Coulby and S. Ward (eds): *The Primary Core National Curriculum*

L. B. Curzon: *Teaching in Further Education* (4th edition)

P. Daunt: *Meeting Disability: A European Response*

J. Freeman: *Gifted Children Growing Up*

J. Nias, G. Southworth and R. Yeomans: *Staff Relationships in the Primary School*

R. Ritchie (ed.): *Profiling in Primary Schools*

A. Rogers: *Adults Learning for Development*

B. Spiecker and R. Straughan (eds): *Freedom and Indoctrination in Education: International Perspectives*

R. Straughan: *Beliefs, Behaviour and Education*

M. Styles, E. Bearne and V. Watson (eds): *After Alice: Exploring Children's Literature*

S. Tann: *Developing Language in the Primary Classroom*

H. Thomas: *Education Costs and Performance*

H. Thomas with G. Kirkpatrick and E. Nicholson: *Financial Delegation and the Local Management of Schools*

D. Thyer and J. Maggs: *Teaching Mathematics to Young Children* (3rd edition)

M. Watts: *The Science of Problem-Solving*

M. Watts (ed.): *Science in the National Curriculum*

J. Wilson: *A New Introduction to Moral Education*

S. Wolfendale *et al.* (eds): *The Profession and Practice of Educational Psychology: Future Directions*

Contents

This book is dedicated to our patients
and their families

About the Authors

Counsellors in the rapidly expanding field of AIDS counselling have until now concentrated on how to help affected individuals. During the period in which the HIV pandemic has been upon us – only ten years – there have been exciting developments in the whole field of counselling and psychotherapy. This is particularly so in our understanding of how the family and community group to which the sufferer belongs interacts with and affects the patient, while the patient in turn has a profound effect on his system. The therapist, too, becomes part of the interacting system.

   Robert Bor, Riva Miller and Eleanor Goldman, as well as having professional training as psychologist, social worker and physician respectively, have grasped the nettle of systemic thinking and have trained and practised as family therapists. In this book they put their profound understanding of this body of knowledge and their skill as counsellors at the service of the AIDs patient, his or her family and intimate friends. Detailed accounts of sessions will help others to improve their own understanding and skills and will encourage them to widen their perspective.

Dr Dora Black
Consultant Child and Adolescent Psychiatrist, Royal Free Hospital, London
July 1992

Robert Bor is both a clinical and a counselling psychologist who has worked in both psychiatric and medical settings. He trained in the practice and teaching of family therapy at the Tavistock Clinic. His experience in HIV work was gained at the Royal Free Hospital, where he worked as a counsellor for five years until 1991. His training and experience have led to his recent interest in the application of systemic thinking to HIV-associated problems. He now lectures in counselling psychology at the City University, London, and is an Honorary Lecturer in Medicine at the Royal Free Hospital School of Medicine. He is co-editor of the international journal *AIDS Care* and a clinical teacher at the Institute of Family Therapy in London. He has undertaken HIV counselling consultancies in the UK and abroad, and is a Churchill Fellow.

Riva Miller has a background in medical social work. She trained as a family therapist at the Tavistock Clinic, at the Institute of Family Therapy and with the Milan Associates in Italy. At present she is a counsellor and family therapist in the Haemophilia Centre and HIV Counselling Co-ordinator for the Royal Free Hospital. She is an Honorary Senior Lecturer in the Royal Free Hospital School of Medicine. She has a consultancy at the North London Blood Transfusion Centre, has acted as an adviser for the World Health Organization, for which she has co-ordinated many workshops on HIV counselling, and is a clinical teacher at the Institute of Family Therapy. She maintains links with family therapy colleagues at the Kensington Consultation Centre, where she works in private practice.

Eleanor Goldman trained as a physician and worked in a variety of medical settings in South Africa before coming to the UK. Since 1976 she has been responsible for the medical care and genetic counselling of patients with inherited bleeding disorders at the Royal Free Hospital Haemophilia Centre. Working with patients and their families led to formal training in family therapy at the Institute of Family Therapy and the Tavistock Clinic. The techniques of family therapy, particularly those of the Milan Associates, have been adapted for both genetic and HIV counselling for families with bleeding disorders.

The three authors are connected through both their similarities and their differences. The similarities lie in their common background of training in systemic family therapy and subsequent application of these principles to work with people affected by HIV disease. The differences in their original professional training have enabled them to form a multidisciplinary team. They have been able to introduce some of these ideas into their own domains of work, starting with the Haemophilia Centre, then into the HIV Service, and to the teaching of counselling.

Foreword

It is a great pleasure to be asked to write a foreword for *Theory and Practice of HIV Counselling: A Systemic Approach*. In my role as Consultant to the HIV counselling programme at the Royal Free Hospital over several years, I was able to watch the exciting development of the ideas described in this latest book, as the story of HIV/AIDS gradually unfolded. It was apparent that the application of systemic thinking and practice provided the authors, their professional colleagues and their patients with a relevant tool with which to address the complex, multisystemic and multifaceted aspects of work with HIV.

In this book, the authors succeed in elaborating clearly and concisely the theoretical underpinnings of the systemic approach, and convey the fundamentally important message that the counsellor should aim to remain curious at all times, exploring together with the patient his experiences, hopes and expectations, avoiding where possible acting on the counsellor's own assumptions, prejudices and beliefs. They illustrate their work throughout with clinical vignettes and extracts from conversations, which allow the reader to study in detail the techniques of questioning which form the basis of the method.

In covering the whole range of work encountered in the field of HIV – the general issues applying to counselling in life-threatening conditions, such as the management of secrecy and confidentiality, as well as the specific issues of pre- and post-test counselling, laboratory tests and clinical trials and the worried well, and the particular clinical problems raised by patients at different stages of the life-cycle (parents, children and adolescents) – the authors enable the reader to share their experiences in managing this challenging and ever-expanding field.

Most importantly, the book conveys a message of hope and the conviction that everyone can be enabled to find a positive aspect to their life even when facing illness and death.

Caroline Lindsey
Consultant Child and Adolescent Psychiatrist,
Tavistock Clinic, London

Preface

The ideas described in this book are the culmination of nearly a decade's experience of counselling people with HIV disease and other medical conditions. Although the authors have been trained in different professions, they are linked by their theoretical approach in counselling. It is beyond the scope of this book to teach the whole of systemic family therapy; nevertheless, we hope to provide an introduction to the concept.

In the authors' view, there is very little difference between counselling and psychotherapy. Counselling is a process by which the counsellor elicits and gives information in such a way that a therapeutic effect is achieved. It may be provided by highly trained specialist counsellors who work in a specific way or in a specific field. HIV counselling may also be the task of health care workers in the course of their work. On the other hand, different conceptual approaches to the evolution, maintenance and resolution of human problems can be distinguished from one another, irrespective of whether these are applied in working with individuals, couples, families, groups or people in organizations. We use the term 'patient' rather than 'client' or 'counsellee' to refer to these people because we work in hospital and clinic settings. This should not be taken to mean that the person is necessarily physically ill.

A systems approach often implies counselling families. The word 'family' denotes both blood relationships and acquired or social relationships. Same-sex relationships are therefore included in this definition of the family. The personal pronoun 'he' rather than 'he/she' has been used throughout the book for counsellors and patients. This does not reflect any bias on the part of the authors but is merely a convenient pronoun.

Acknowledgements

We are grateful to our colleagues Heather Salt, Derval Murray and Isobel Scher, who helped us to develop and extend our theoretical ideas. Their interest and support have enabled us to bring clarity to our counselling approach.

Many of our ideas about systemic thinking have come from our training in family therapy. Our colleagues at the Child and Family Department of the Tavistock Clinic, the Institute of Family Therapy (London) and the Milan Centre for the Study of the Family have, at different stages, contributed to our understanding and clinical application of systemic theory.

We are indebted to a number of colleagues, both physicians and administrators, who enabled us to apply our counselling approach. Dr Peter Kernoff and Dr Christine Lee, of the Royal Free Hospital Katherine Domandy Haemophilia Centre and Haemostasis Unit, enabled us to introduce the ideas described in this book into the hospital. Mr John Cooper, Chief Executive of the Royal Free Hampstead, NHS Trust, and his staff, gave us support and encouragement to set up the District HIV/AIDS Counselling Unit. Dr Margaret Johnson, Consultant in HIV, has extended our practice to her in- and outpatients units. Dr Jonathan Elford of the Royal Free Hospital School of Medicine supported us in our research pursuits.

Naomi Roth, our editor at Cassell, offered support and encouragement at all stages of the preparation of this book.

PART ONE

THEORY OF SYSTEMIC HIV COUNSELLING

ONE

Introduction and Overview

'What is the use of a book', thought Alice, 'without pictures or conversations?'

Lewis Carroll

Confidentiality prevents us from publishing pictures, but we have recorded many conversations. Names have been altered to preserve the anonymity of the individuals concerned. We hope that these may serve to illustrate some of the dilemmas faced by those infected with HIV and by others in the systems which they inhabit – family, lovers, medical workers and counsellors, to name but a few. They also demonstrate how solutions can sometimes be found through open communication.

Since AIDS was first recognized as a new health problem in the USA in 1981, counsellors and other professionals have been at the forefront of care-giving to people infected with or affected by HIV. Alongside the rapid advances over the decade in the fields of epidemiology, virology, immunology, clinical management, nursing care, clinical therapy and prophylaxis, there has been a supreme effort to understand more about the psychosocial sequelae of HIV disease and to translate that comprehension into counselling. A wide range of professionals recognize that counselling is not new to their work. However, recent emphasis on HIV counselling and the apparent special features this may encompass may affect how some people view the counselling task. Some have trained to become specialist HIV counsellors whilst for others it has meant taking another look at their counselling skills and enhancing them. For the majority of professionals, a basic competence in HIV counselling may be sufficient to help them identify and manage patient problems in the course of their work. This experience can, in turn, enable them to feel more confident in talking to patients about sensitive issues such as sex, sexuality, disfigurement, death, dying, bereavement and social stigma. We have written not only for experienced counsellors who have an interest in developing their skills in HIV counselling, but also for the range of other health care providers who manage HIV-related problems in the course of their work.

There is some difference between *being a counsellor* and *having counselling skills*. Many health care professionals have a primary training in medicine, nursing, physiotherapy or other allied professions. Almost all of them counsel in the course of their work. They constantly interact with patients, giving information, clarifying treatment options and helping people to adjust to new, and sometimes unwelcome, circumstances. Specialist counsellors, on the other hand, are usually people who have advanced training in counselling, psychotherapy or family therapy, some of whom may be professionally trained in other disciplines, such as medicine, clinical psychology, nursing or social work. Although specialist training is not a requirement to practise as a counsellor, there are likely to be occasions when any counsellor sees the need to refer a patient to a specialist counsellor in the same way as a doctor may refer medical problems to a specialist colleague. The ideas presented in this book may be of use both to specialist counsellors and others who counsel. When we use the term 'counsellor' in the text, it may apply to any of the professions mentioned.

The special problems that arise in the context of HIV disease management, coupled with time constraints in some clinical settings and the complex dilemmas and powerful feelings invoked by this problem, may challenge people's existing counselling maps. This book attempts to convey one particular map that has been applied and developed in several clinical settings and in relation to a range of social and clinical problems. There are other maps and theories that may be equally relevant.

This volume is a companion text to our previous publication, *AIDS: A Guide to Clinical Counselling* (London: Science Press, 1988). The basic tenets of HIV counselling were set out in that book and an approach to counselling sessions was described. Readers are encouraged to refer to that text for additional information on HIV counselling practice. The ideas set out there have been extended and largely reflect the developments in our counselling and therapeutic approach and style as a result of our continuing experience in this field, the changes in the socio-medical context of HIV disease and the challenging questions about our practice put to us by our colleagues and students. The emphasis on psychological theory, in this case a systems approach, is conveyed in this book.

All models of diagnosis and treatment exist in a theoretical framework. Both assessment and treatment are linked to the counsellor's theoretical ideas. In the traditional medical model of diagnosis, there is an individual orientation which leads one to look for indications of problems *inside* the person and to direct treatment exclusively at the person as the intervention target.

The systemic view considers the reciprocity of relationships. For instance, if something happens to one member of a family, it will affect the rest of the family, whose response, in turn, will affect the behaviour of that individual. This means that behaviour cannot be studied in isolation without taking into account the situation in which it occurs. All behaviour is part of an interactive process whether at home, at work, or in a counselling session. The counsellor may influence the patient whose reactions, in turn, have an effect on the counsellor. Counselling is not a process of 'doing something to someone'. It is best defined as an interaction between the counsellor and the patient, and also includes others such as the patient's family, lovers and friends, and the counsellor's colleagues, as well as members of the health care team. Systemic counsellors address the belief systems which influence the patient's behaviour in the context of his social setting.

The system may be the person with HIV and his family, or it may be the patient and his health carers. The authors, comprising a multidisciplinary team of a clinical psychologist, a social worker and a medical doctor, represent a system. They have different backgrounds but are linked by being family therapists and working in the same hospital setting. A counsellor and an individual client can also represent a system.

Systemic work can be accomplished with an individual by linking him with others in his system, even if they are not present at the interview, by asking hypothetical questions about their views, for example, 'If your girlfriend were here today, what would she say was her greatest concern?'

Systemic thinking crosses cultural boundaries and takes into account religious and ethnic beliefs. Every event has a past and a future and these need to be explored.

Most importantly, systemic counsellors should help the individual and his family to consider the resources they already have and those they might seek out to help them cope. Asking how they have coped with difficulties in the past and hypothetical questions about future coping will link them with others and enable them to acquire different views of their situation.

We have thought a good deal about the tasks of counsellors and some of our beliefs; the contents of the first six chapters describe these more fully. The main beliefs we adhere to and which influence our approach to counselling can be summarized as follows:

- We do not believe that HIV disease inevitably or invariably leads to psychological or social problems for everyone, although problems can arise at different points in the course of illness.

- Medical or physical problems have implications for relationships, whether these are between family members, lovers or health care providers. They can also affect people's view of themselves.

- The 'family' may be the patient's most important social system: it may be a biological or social entity. We do not have predetermined views about relationship constellations; for example, two men in an enduring relationship may be a family. Problems about HIV disease may arise in the context of family relationships and can be resolved within them.

- We have clear goals and objectives for the counselling session, based on systemic theory, which are to define the problem, consider for whom it is a problem and work towards its resolution. However, we do not have fixed ideas about what would be the best solution in a particular case.

- We do not believe that there is only one approach to counselling. Different ideas are healthy and may themselves even be therapeutic. Whichever route one takes, a map is necessary to help to conceptualize problems and their possible resolution. Theory is also important for teaching others about counselling. In some circumstances, counsellors may even have to explain their actions to others in a court of law, and theory may be an important aspect of this. Underdeveloped training in psychological theories or vague theoretical ideas are a recipe for confusion in counselling or therapy sessions and for both confusing and abusing the patient.

• The objective reality of HIV as an illness affects people in different ways. Our task as counsellors is to help patients identify what meaning this illness has for them. We are dealing with ideas and beliefs. As Hoffman (1981, p. 344) states, 'the reality "out there" is unknowable because it changes as we watch, and because our watching changes it.' As counsellors, we continually ask questions of ourselves that help us to understand what assumptions we may be making about people, their relationships and their adjustment to illness. Our concern is to avoid situations in which patients may feel pushed to see things in the way we see them, or where we inadvertently disqualify their ideas or feelings.

We describe a counselling approach as it relates to psychotherapeutic counselling rather than information-giving counselling. The emphasis is on dealing primarily with psychosocial problems as they relate to HIV disease rather than on health education. Our focus is limited to the management of psychological and social problems with a description of a particular theoretical approach. A *problem-focused systemic* counselling approach is useful for several reasons.

1 HIV disease is foremost a medical problem, with psychological, social, political, economic and legal sequelae. It is not inevitably a psychological problem. This counselling approach addresses the multiplicity of problems associated with HIV disease. While a diagnosis of HIV infection can lead to major psychological problems, such as depression, adjustment reaction or an exacerbation of existing problems, these are rarely the main, underlying or enduring problems for people with HIV disease.

2 An overemphasis on psychological care may inadvertently cause some patients to believe they have a *psychological* problem. The counselling approach described in this book starts out with the premise that problems first need to be identified and defined by patients or health care providers. Most psychological problems can be assessed and managed, and in some cases prevented, in the course of comprehensive medical care.

3 Increasing workloads and constraints arising from pressure on time mean that health care providers may need to 'achieve the most' with their patient in the shortest possible time. The conventional fifty-minute psychotherapy session may be mostly inappropriate to HIV management. Brief, problem-focused counselling emphasizes problem identification and resolution. A clearly mapped-out plan of action may itself be a major psychotherapeutic intervention for a patient who is uncertain, anxious or bewildered about his recent diagnosis of HIV infection. Although the number of sessions may be fewer than with conventional psychotherapy, problem-focused counselling can sometimes extend over a longer period, with sessions being held at greater intervals.

4 Patients increasingly expect health care providers not only to be experts in their chosen field such as medicine, nursing, laboratory science or social

work, but also to have the sensitivity and skills to discuss complex treatment and care issues. The systemic approach attaches importance to conversational and problem-solving skills.

5 The counselling skills described can be applied to general problem-solving. Counsellors can never be taught 'what-to-say-when' in any psychotherapeutic approach. Systemic counselling introduces the concept of a 'map' for problem-solving. There are clearly set out procedures in the counselling map and these can be easily adapted to fit with most psychotherapeutic approaches, including client-centred, cognitive and psychodynamic ones, and in response to a wide range of problems which patients may describe.

Skills for counselling people with HIV disease may be of use to the majority of health care providers worldwide as this can help them to address some of their patients' problems. Although our experience has been gained in a developed country with relatively good health and social services, we feel that the model could equally be adapted and applied in other settings where there may be poverty, deprivation and minimal medical care. At the same time it is important to note that counselling has its origins in a Western ethic of informed consent and an approach to mental health care. Psychotherapy and counselling imply weekly, or more frequent, sessions with a trained therapist over many years. While this may be necessary for some people who have HIV disease, open-ended psychotherapy or counselling for personal development can be distinguished from brief counselling as (a) the latter is often problem-focused; (b) it may include advice-giving or the provision of information; (c) the identified patient may not have symptoms of psychopathology *per se*; and (d) counselling need not continue over many sessions. Both approaches may be used in caring for people with HIV disease, provided there has first been a comprehensive assessment of the problem in the light of the stage of the patient's illness.

The systemic approach guides the professional in taking a neutral view of problems and solutions (see Chapter 2). The counselling conversation is facilitated by asking interventive and therapeutic questions. Assumptions on the part of the counsellor about the nature of reactions to a diagnosis may impede rather than facilitate the patient's management. Where counsellors have fixed views about how people should adapt to an HIV diagnosis, apparent resistance and denial may become the focus of sessions as counsellors and their patients 'compete' to assert their views and beliefs.

We have chosen to address certain ideas and themes of counselling theory and practice as they relate to HIV disease in the full knowledge that it would require a much larger text to cover every aspect of HIV counselling. The book is divided into three parts: the first part (Chapters 1 to 6) describes the theory behind the systemic approach to counselling. The processes of problem definition and problem resolution are addressed, drawing on examples from our clinical work. The second part (Chapters 7 to 16) covers the application of the theory to a range of clinical issues and problems such as counselling for an HIV antibody test, counselling about laboratory tests and drug trials, and managing secrecy-related problems.

Approaches to counselling the worried well, the terminally ill and the bereaved are also covered. Some of the emerging specialities in HIV counselling, such as counselling women, children and adolescents, are addressed. We have deliberately excluded special reference to counselling people from traditional 'risk groups' – such as gay men and intravenous drug users – because with the increasing spread of HIV, it is invidious to single out risk groups and perpetuate stereotypes. Problem-focused counselling should be applicable to any counselling situation. Finally, there is a chapter on the clinical aspects of HIV infection, which has been contributed by Dr Bertle Squire and Dr Margaret Johnson from the HIV Unit at the Royal Free Hospital, London. In this chapter, the authors describe the evolving biomedical context of HIV disease and discuss some of the trends anticipated for the 1990s. These might have implications for the nature of the psychosocial problems that patients may experience and how they may be dealt with.

The main theme addressed in these chapters is the psychological care of those affected by HIV. We have deliberately chosen not to discuss the care and support of professional staff because this was described in our previous book. Nonetheless, investment in staff support and personal development will contribute to better standards of care for patients and their families.

The idea of a map may be a fitting metaphor for these ideas. The theory, ideas and techniques can help to guide professionals in counselling. There is not only one map for any territory. The context or nature of problems differs between settings, patients and counsellors: additionally, the territory itself keeps changing. Advances in biomedicine and changes in the social or political circumstances of those with HIV disease, as well as changes in the spread of HIV, may pose enormous challenges to patients and health care providers. Counselling and psychotherapy can be very complex activities and people are trained for many years. Some ideas may be useful and relevant to readers; some may not fit with others. Either way, the task as we see it is to help counsellors and patients to look differently, and more critically, at what they are currently thinking and doing, and also to confirm some of their own ideas. After all, this is what we do in counselling or psychotherapy.

TWO

Systemic Theory and Practice in Counselling People with HIV Disease

In thinking about the world we are faced with the same kind of problem as the cartographer who tries to cover the curved face of the earth with a sequence of plane maps. We can only expect an approximate representation of reality from such a procedure, and all rational knowledge is therefore necessarily limited.

Fritjof Capra

INTRODUCTION

An important feature of skilful counselling is an ability to approach each new case and problem with a receptive openness and to recognize that, where relevant, each patient will require different therapeutic approaches and procedures. This needs to be balanced with a level of competence in tried and tested therapeutic approaches and interventions. Some aspects of systemic theory that relate to the practice of counselling patients with HIV disease are set out in this chapter.

THE MAIN TENETS OF A SYSTEMS APPROACH

The essential features of a systems approach are:

1 *Behaviour and problems occur in a context.* That is, they should be examined and understood in the milieu in which they arise. Systemic counsellors subscribe to the ideas of Watzlawick, Beavin and Jackson (1967) with regard to the basic axioms of communication. These are: (a) one cannot *not* communicate; (b) every communication tells us something about a relationship; and (c) communication always includes ideas about content (*what* is being said) and process (*how* it is said and what this conveys).

2 *There is reciprocity in relationships.* If something happens to an individual it will have an impact on other people and may affect how they behave in

response to new behaviour or beliefs: 'at the heart of all psychosocial enquiry, for clinicians and researchers alike, is the focus on interaction. In the arena of chronic illness one's concern is the interaction of a disease with an individual, family or other biopsychosocial systems' (Rolland, 1984, p. 246). The resolution of emotional problems may, for example, create a new problem for an ill person as his friends may no longer feel the need to visit him as often. This may result in his feeling more lonely. While much work in systemic counselling has focused on the family, counsellors also work with individuals, couples and groups. New ideas and beliefs that arise in these contexts may have a 'knock-on' effect on other family members, thereby affecting the family as a whole.

3 *Relationships between people (whether they are family members or colleagues) are punctuated by beliefs and behaviours.* New ideas or beliefs can lead to different behaviours and vice versa. There may be, for example, a belief that people with HIV disease must see a professional for psychological support. Some patients may then feel that they have both a physical and an emotional problem. Patients who attend for counselling but who do not discuss problems may be seen by some counsellors to be 'denying' problems. Behaviour, thought and emotion are interdependent. Counsellors or therapists can intervene with patients with respect to either their behaviour or their ideas and beliefs. Systems practitioners tend to focus their interventions on ideas and beliefs.

4 *Problems may occur at particular developmental stages of individuals or families.* Problems are most likely to arise at points of change or transition, such as when children are born, when young adults prepare to leave home, and when a family member becomes ill or dies. Transitions constantly occur in life, and these may be more frequent in people with HIV disease. If these changes threaten the stability of the family system, some members may

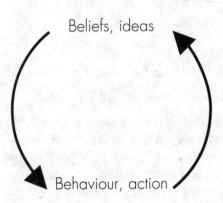

Beliefs, ideas

Behaviour, action

attempt to restrain other individuals and the family as a whole from changing. This is often characterized by rigid interactional behaviour. Psychopathology or symptomatic behaviour in an individual family member may develop as a consequence of these tensions within the family. This serves to restrain the family system from growing or developing and therefore acts to maintain the equilibrium or homeostasis of the family. Psychological symptoms signal rigidity and distress in the family system, but are not necessarily the main or underlying problem (Andolfi *et al.*, 1983). Symptoms usually indicate relationship problems. A child in a family who bed-wets or steals, for example, may have become unsettled as a result of problems in the relationship between his parents. Similarly depression in one partner may reflect anxiety about the spouse having an extra-marital affair.

5 *Problems may also occur when reality is denied.* A patient with HIV may, for example, be denying reality when he becomes unexpectedly unwell, but will not allow others to take care of him when this is appropriate and necessary. Someone who demands complete certainty and predictability in life may also be at increased risk of developing psychological problems, as the nature of this disease is that much is unknown and therefore there are many uncertainties.

6 *There is reciprocity in the counselling setting.* Counselling is not a process of 'doing-something-to-someone'. It is best defined as a dialogue between the counsellor and the patient. Feedback must constantly be evaluated and processed. People are affected by wider political and economic systems. For example, if a hospital is unable to offer a particular specialized treatment, this will influence patient care. Providers of health care may then have to deal with the frustration and anger of patients who feel that they are not being offered the full range of possible treatments.

7 *HIV disease is a medical problem of great complexity.* It is expected that problems will arise for patients which will have implications for relationships with family members, friends and professionals, among others. It is impossible to have consensus about all aspects of care because staff, patients and ideas in medical science are constantly changing.

8 *Problems that present to counsellors are generally expressed in language and in the course of a conversation.* Counselling is mostly engaging in a conversation about a problem. Systems theory has contributed significantly to insights into language, problems and solutions.

Empathy

A hallmark of counselling practice, particularly from the point of view of the 'client-centred approach' (Rogers, 1951), has been the importance of empathy in the counselling relationship. Empathy is conveyed in two different ways in counselling. Listening to the patient, respecting his views and attempting to understand his predicament or problem more fully is one description of empathy. The counsellor is also being empathic when he moves at the rate or pace that the patient dictates. If the counsellor introduces ideas to the patient before he is ready to accept them, the counsellor is imposing his views and potentially making assumptions about the patient. It has been suggested that a counsellor's warm and empathic style facilitates problem-solving. Undoubtedly, the counsellor's sensitivity, interest in the patient's problems and concern for his physical condition are important if the counselling relationship is to develop. However, empathy and listening alone are unlikely fully to satisfy the patient's expressed need for change (Branwhite, 1991).

Some professionals caring for people with HIV disease may not feel able to convey the same empathy to their patients in all aspects of their problems. Everyone has some prejudices and preconceived ideas about right and wrong. These may relate to a patient's lifestyle or to the patient's problem. Training and supervision can help counsellors to identify their prejudices and deal with them in the counselling setting. However, some may never feel empathic towards people with certain problems. The counsellor may come to understand the complex nature and circumstances of some problems, such as child sex abuse or domestic violence, but feel uncomfortable counselling either their perpetrators or victims. In situations where the counsellor's own prejudices impede the therapy, we recommend that the counsellor refers the patient to a colleague. Ongoing disagreements with the patient, feeling ineffective in helping him or personal distaste for the patient's lifestyle, whatever this may be, should signal to the counsellor that he needs to seek supervision or refer the patient elsewhere.

Systems theory and ideas about diagnosis and assessment

Moving to a systemic view, the counsellor invites the individual to think about the family and other relationships, and to bring them to sessions, where appropriate. The counsellor looks beyond the individual to his relationships with other systems, such as the family, for indications of the problem. All forms of diagnosis and therapy involve asking questions that result in disclosure of the relevant information to the counsellor. Questions form an integral part of the process of diagnosis, which in turn is inseparable from the process of counselling. The process of diagnosis is not merely a procedure for labelling, for this by itself may be destructive. Rather it is seen as an ongoing process of observing, examining and clarifying a stated problem within its whole context. The aim is to formulate appropriate methods of dealing with that problem. *Diagnosis* is a continual process which evolves with treatment.

The Milan Team, led by the Italian psychiatrist Mara Selvini-Palazzoli, introduced the circular interview as a means for conducting a systemic investigation of the changes and differences in family relationships which recursively support dysfunctional interactions or symptoms in the family (Selvini-Palazzoli *et al.*, 1980b). The development of an hypothesis about the family's relational patterns and the circular interaction among family members that leads to the occurrence of the system is a central procedure in this assessment process, and is described below.

HYPOTHESIZING

What is a systemic 'hypothesis'?

In order to guide the counsellor in this problem-defining task, he needs to develop an *hypothesis*, or calculated guess, about the problem and what it may mean. This is more fully described in our book *AIDS: A Guide to Clinical Counselling*. Hypotheses are composite ideas about a family's functioning and relationship patterns with respect to a symptom or problem. The Milan Team who first described the use of systemic hypotheses in counselling (Selvini-Palazzoli *et al.*, 1980b) were not concerned about the *truths* of the counsellor's explanations or ideas, but rather the *usefulness* of their formulations. In an attempt to furnish an answer to the question of whether there is one true hypothesis, Hoffman (1981, p. 294) wrote that 'there are as many possibilities of the truth as there are places from which to stand and look at it'.

To make the systemic hypothesis meaningful, the counsellor needs to look to a range of relationships and factors outside the clinical interview and to include ideas about the individual and the family's stages of life development, the stage of HIV disease and the views of the referrer (Selvini-Palazzoli *et al.*, 1980a). The systemic counsellor is also interested in incorporating different people's *perceptions* of problems into an hypothesis in order to identify the best way to address and resolve the problem. An example of an hypothesis might be:

> Dr Grey has asked me to see this patient because the patient seems depressed. It may be that the patient is becoming more unwell and that from a medical point of view, there is less that the medical team can offer the patient. The patient may seem more depressed because he has not yet told his family that he has HIV for a fear of upsetting them. Consequently, he may feel more lonely and isolated. He may also be anxious about his condition and feel that the doctors and nurses are not talking to him as openly as they were previously. Maybe everyone thinks that a counsellor will 'cheer the patient up' but not upset him. In this way, it seems that the belief is 'support and protect everyone emotionally, but don't upset people by talking about what might happen to the patient in the future'.

Hypotheses reflect the counsellor's view of reality rather than what is 'really' occurring and they are used to guide the counsellor and keep a focus on the problem and what it may mean. They are revised within sessions, as new information comes to light, and between sessions. Labelling or placing a patient in a psychiatric diagnostic category tends to fix him in a single reality. For this reason, a systemic hypothesis that addresses the problem and its context may be more appropriate, particularly in dealing with the problem of HIV disease, which may have significant personal and interpersonal consequences.

Constructing an hypothesis

The construction of an hypothesis involves making use of all available information to create a therapeutic *reality*. The hypothesis should be *circular and relational*, which means that all information gathered in the session relevant to a symptom should be used to create a new view or understanding of that symptom in the context of family relationships. It is through the process of *questioning*, which is described below, that the ideas in the hypothesis will be put to the test, leading to either confirmation or some revision of the original hypothesis. Revision of the hypothesis in accordance with feedback from the clinical interview proceeds throughout the course of counselling.

Hypothesizing is similar to what Bateson (1979) viewed as a process of weaving several levels of abstraction. One begins with the observed data, including behaviour or statements, then on a more abstract level one links the behaviour with ideas and beliefs to form a map of the situation. The patient's expression of feelings in the session or reports of behaviour, incidents or feelings are important insofar as they help to contribute to an understanding of his problems, his context and the ideas or beliefs that are associated with his problems. In order not to make assumptions about feelings or behaviour, the counsellor needs to enquire about what these may signal or mean in relation to the problem. The counsellor should also check other family members' ideas about these in order to obtain a more complete and systemic view. The counsellor is interested in the relevant history of the patient and the problem, but only as it throws light on *how* things have come to be as they are, and the *ideas and beliefs* that are generated around the evolution and maintenance of the problem. This is conceptually different from a line of enquiry which attempts to answer the question, 'What went wrong to cause this problem?'

The use of a genogram, as described in Chapter 16 (pages 152–4), is an effective method of introducing themes of loss, mourning, adaptation and coping to counselling sessions.

CIRCULAR QUESTIONS

The counsellor's interview with the patient is an important source of information: 'a clinical interview affords far more opportunities to act therapeutically than most people realize' (Tomm, 1987a, p. 3). Counselling conversations are not ordinary conversations as there is the potential for emotional pain and healing for patients (Tomm, 1988).

Circularity, as opposed to linear cause–effect reasoning, is a hallmark of the systemic counsellor. The counsellor conducts the session using feedback from the family about relationships and interactive patterns (Selvini-Palazzoli *et al.*, 1980b). In the traditional medical model, symptomatic behaviour or psychopathology may be seen to be caused by biological changes or repressed events (psychodynamic view). Irrespective of the source or cause of the problem, the medical model focuses on the *individual* who is seen as the *locus of pathology*. Investigations proceed along a linear course, linking past events to symptoms.

When the technique of circular questioning is used, the process of the interview itself will reflect circular thinking. Thus, the underlying philosophy and methods used to conduct the process of diagnosis and treatment are congruent. Questions are the main catalyst for patient change and healing and they provide patients with opportunities to make further choices in their lives. There is a wide range of questions that can be used in counselling. Linear questions, sometimes termed 'closed questions', usually require a 'yes' or 'no' reply from the patient and are helpful if information or content is required by the counsellor. The term 'circular questions' applies to the range of interventive or therapeutic questions that are used in addition to linear questions in systemic counselling. Some examples of questions are set out below:

Linear question	Do you get depressed easily?
Future-oriented question	How do you see John managing if he were to become unwell?
Relationship question	Which of your parents gets more upset when they think that Sue may never have children?
Difference question	Is it more or less stressful for you to carry on without having an HIV test, but worrying about it, or having a test and maybe having to deal with a positive test result?
Circular question	What might happen to you in your relationship with your sister if neither of your parents was able to carry on looking after her?
Reflexive question (commenting on process)	Who takes care of your mother at home when she cries and is upset as she is now?

Using the process of circular questioning (Selvini-Palazzoli *et al.*, 1980b) the counsellor is able to track very closely not only relationship patterns in the present, but any shifts in allegiances at the time the problem first appeared. The basic tenet is always to ask questions that address a *difference* or *define a relationship*: for example: 'Who is most worried about Steven's problem?' or 'What does your mother do when your father gets very upset?' One aim of circular questioning is to complete all the circuits in the system and to cross-reference information. Another aim is to find out when in the family's development important coalitions changed and how this may have become a problem for the family (Penn, 1982). At the same time the use of this technique inserts punctuation that emphasizes difference and circularity while connecting the counsellor and all members of the family.

Some advantages of using questions

- If asked in a sensitive manner, questions may seem less confrontational than statements and less unsettling than lengthy periods of silence.
- Asking questions defines the counsellor as being interested in the patient's views. This may help the counsellor to guard against becoming prescriptive.
- The answers to some questions and the manner in which they are answered may provide important diagnostic material for the counsellor.

– Questions are a useful way of dealing with sensitive issues with patients or where there may be resistance to change.
– Questions are also a powerful source of engagement between the counsellor and family members throughout the course of counselling.
– The counsellor may feel less under pressure to offer solutions; some of this responsibility is transferred to the patient through the use of questions.
– Questions help to reveal something about the ideas and beliefs of the patient, which are central to this approach to counselling. Through the use of circular questions and the information they elicit, the perception of the problem by the patient and his family members will become evident, including points of agreement and disagreement.
– Some questions may be phrased in such a way that new connections between people and ideas are made which help patients to view problems in a different light. Simply hearing the questions, which may convey new ideas or connections, can be therapeutic for the patient.

Because they are grounded in the ideas of circularity, recursiveness, feedback and difference, circular questions can be used to explore different perceptions and views of relationships. They are designed to help patients to view their situation, whatever it may be, in a different way. They provide the patient and his family with the opportunity to view themselves in the context of relationships in an interacting system. This extended view may in turn lead to new ideas about a problem and its resolution. Hypothetical or future-oriented questions are particularly effective in this regard. Combining the concept of future and change simultaneously through future questions addresses and challenges the system's capacity to evolve. This makes it more difficult for the family system to maintain its current patterns of ideas or behaviours. Questions can also address the historical and developmental contexts of the family (Fleuridas, Nelson and Rosenthal, 1986). There is no such thing as a 'wrong' question, although certain questions will be more useful than others; everything the counsellor 'does or says, or chooses not to do or not to say, can be thought of as an intervention that could be therapeutic, nontherapeutic or countertherapeutic' (Tomm, 1987a, p. 5). The questions that the counsellor asks help to construct a therapeutic reality. This reality in turn enables the counsellor to formulate a particular intervention, or the introduction of this new reality may become an intervention in itself.

The Milan Team have continued to describe several methods by which relationship information can be gathered. The focus is on 'difference' questions. For example: 'Who gets most upset when your son has to go into hospital?' or 'If Paul were to need more support, who in the family would most be in a position to provide this?' While the content of the conversation is of importance, so too are the reactions in the session of all of the family members to the responses. Hoffman (1981, p. 301) pointed out three implications of the method:

> First of all, such questions make people stop and think, rather than react in a stereotypical way. The people who are not talking also listen attentively. Secondly, these questions cut into escalations and fights, not only between

family members, but between a therapist and family members. And thirdly, they seem to trigger more of the same kind of 'difference' thinking which is essentially circular because it introduces the ideas of links made up of shifting perspectives.

Asking questions of those in the session is also useful for bypassing 'stuckness' in counselling and uncovering the relevance of interconnectedness of different people and their ideas. The connections and comments on behaviour and perceptions through circular questions open up discussion about behaviour, beliefs, feelings and the future. All of these are crucial to counselling people with HIV disease or who are affected by it. Most important of all, circular questions can introduce new information and punctuate reality. This cannot easily be done through linear questions that focus on unravelling the 'truth'. When circular questions no longer help to provide information relevant to the hypothesis or to the generation of new hypotheses, the counsellor may have lost a sense of curiosity (Cecchin, 1987), and it is at this point that supervision or consultation may be most appropriate and helpful (Bor and Miller, 1990).

INTERVENING THERAPEUTICALLY

Some of the reasons for conducting the clinical interview through the use of questions have been set out above. It should be clear that questions are asked of the patient and family members in order to: (a) elicit information by checking all views and not making any assumptions; (b) establish relational patterns; (c) clarify ideas and beliefs; (d) help prevent the counsellor from becoming drawn into the pattern of the problem; and (e) act as a conceptual and executive tool, to guide the counsellor in the counselling session by constantly using feedback to revise his hypothesis. In our experience, circular questioning has a special place in counselling people with HIV disease and is one of our main therapeutic techniques.

A central theme in counselling people with HIV disease is to help them to face loss or the potential for loss. The individual and family need to create a meaning for the illness that can help to preserve their sense of competence, which includes their belief about how they will support the HIV-infected family member and influence events (Rolland, 1990). These beliefs are wide-ranging, but may include ideas about whether there is hope, from a medical point of view, or whether the course of illness can in any way be shifted. Blame or guilt about infection with HIV may be invoked by some beliefs, which may be so powerful that they overshadow beliefs about the illness and its consequences. If a belief emerges that a son who has contracted the disease through his homosexual practices is blamed by his parents for his illness, then each stage in the course of his illness will be highlighted by his parents' anger and blame, thereby potentially ignoring some of the patient's physical and psychological needs.

In some situations, beliefs about blame, responsibility and guilt may serve to 'deflect' family members from the overwhelming emotional pain of losing a child. The pain may be in relation to 'separation anxiety, existential aloneness, denial, sadness, disappointment, anger, resentment, guilt, exhaustion and desperation' (Rolland, 1990, p. 230). The feelings may be both intense and ambivalent; there may be a desire to be closely and deeply connected with a family member and, at the same time, a need to escape from the emotional pain and a longing to feel disconnected from the person and the problem. Furthermore, these painful feelings about loss may have to be endured in secret and in isolation because of the social stigma associated with HIV disease. *Coping with living with HIV disease may be as difficult for the family as coping with the actual death.* The anticipation of the loss through physical illness can so disturb the current functioning of each member of the family, as well as the family as a whole, that the counsellor may need to address the present in the context of the future. In order to be systemic and to create a circular view, the counsellor would need to address the present in the context of the past and the future in the context of the past. An important task of the counsellor is *to push the family system forwards in order that individuals do not become stuck* at a particular point in their development. The counsellor has the task of laying the foundation for the family's future and for future counselling, which may include bereavement counselling. A loss, through death, is possibly the most profound of the losses addressed in the course of counselling and the principles for dealing with other problems in counselling are very similar since many psychological problems arise in relation to difficulty with change, which implies some loss.

Counselling people about dying and loss is but one aspect of the problem, and the counsellor should also address the other aspects of this, i.e. problems with living, with the patient and family. This approach is described more fully in Chapter 6. Families in which there is chronic illness may 'have difficulty imagining their future because of its potential loss or deterioration. They can lose the systemic flexibility that allows the future to hold new meanings' (Penn, 1985, p. 305). The counsellor can help family members to face the uncertainty of the future and the pain of the present by enhancing their capacity to acknowledge the possibility of loss, but at the same time to sustain a measure of hope that will help them to carry on.

From a systemic point of view, the use of circular and future-oriented questions can help to achieve some of these goals. Future-oriented questions help the family to talk about the future, their fears about what may happen to each person or to the family as a whole, and provide information to the counsellor about how the family sees itself both in the present and in the future, with or without the member with HIV. Where the counsellor has the impression that the family has no view of or hope for the future, these questions can trigger the creation of a sense of or a belief about the future by family members. Some examples of these questions are:

> How do you see the next six months in this family knowing that Raymond has HIV?
>
> If things did not go in the way in which you had hoped and Raymond became unwell sooner than you had expected, who might be most upset? How might

their being upset show? How do you think that this may affect your parents' relationship?

These questions address perceptions of the future, fears of a deterioration in health and the impact of these on relationships. Perhaps the greatest difficulty that counsellors face when trying out this approach for the first time is to know what questions to ask. As previously stated, some questions are more useful than others. Counsellors should be motivated by their interest and curiosity; each time they think they have become clear about an issue they should ask more questions that help them to understand the problem from a different angle. It often happens in counselling that the counsellor addresses only one implication of a problem; for example, how it presents. The counsellor should remind himself that the implications of a problem for relationships and the beliefs that these may generate should also be addressed.

Training and supervision are required in all counselling approaches for acquiring skills and developing expertise. Some readers may also want to learn more about the approach and techniques described in this chapter and they should consult the references cited. The following additional references set out how to learn to use questions therapeutically: Feinberg, 1990: Fleuridas, Nelson and Rosenthal, 1986; and Mauksch and Roesler, 1990.

THREE

Exploring and Defining Problems in HIV Counselling

*Alice ... went on. 'Would you tell me, please, which way I ought to
go from here?'*
'That depends a good deal on where you want to get to,' said the Cat.

Lewis Carroll

A clear definition of 'the problem' is required by the counsellor before he
introduces any other intervention. This is an integral part of counselling and
psychotherapeutic practice, and not merely an assessment phase. It provides an
opportunity to place a frame around a systemic hypothesis and gather information
which is used to refine the hypothesis. The extent to which counselling will be
successful depends, in part, on the way in which it begins and, therefore, how the
problem is defined. Having started a conversation with a patient, some counsellors
may be uncertain as to what to say next or where to lead the conversation. This
chapter describes how the patient's problem can be clarified and defined.

WHAT IS THE CONTEXT OF THE PROBLEM?

For counsellors fully to understand the definition of the problem, they may require
answers to certain key questions. The first of these may be to identify the context in
which the problem is defined. The following possibilities, as shown in Table 3.1,
should be considered (Van Trommel, 1983, p. 77).

Table 3.1   Defining the Problem

THE CONTEXT OF THE PROBLEM	EXAMPLE
1 The problem presented is related to the family system of the patient.	The parents of a man with HIV see the illness of their son as just punishment for his being homosexual.

2 The problem presented is related to other living systems of the patient.	The employer of an HIV-infected woman has decided to terminate her employment.
3 The problem presented is related to other therapeutic systems with which the patient maintains contact.	A health adviser in a sexually transmitted diseases clinic thinks that a patient, who has HIV, 'is denying his illness and needs to work through his anger towards his boyfriend, in order to come to terms with his situation'.
4 The problem presented is related to the system within which the counsellor works.	A consultant refers a patient to an HIV counsellor to help the patient maintain hope even though his health is declining. He is asking the counsellor to undertake this formidable task because he cannot face giving 'bad news' to the patient.

These contexts can be explored by the counsellor asking some of the following questions of himself during a session:

> How long has the patient had the problem?
>
> When did it start?
>
> Why is the patient talking about it now?
>
> How does it affect the patient emotionally and physically?
>
> How does the problem present?
>
> Who else *should* be involved?
>
> Who else knows about the problem?
>
> Is this a problem that requires counselling, or is it better dealt with by another professional?

Patients will sometimes describe a catalogue of problems which may overwhelm the counsellor. The patient should then be asked to rank the problems in order of severity so that the most pressing problems can be tackled first. This helps both the counsellor and patient to feel that the situation is manageable. The patient can also be helped to feel that it is acceptable to have problems. Assigning priority to problems helps the patient and counsellor to view them in relation to one another and therefore introduces a new view or reframe of the problems.

The counsellor's choice of language is important, and complex issues may need to be simplified so as to be meaningful to patients. Using language that fits with that of the patient and checking that the meaning of words used are understood may prevent misunderstandings or assumptions being made. Anxiety, for example, is frequently expressed in general and non-specific terms by patients. Counsellors may find it useful to help the patient to convey how he feels by asking him to describe behaviours. It is easier to consider therapeutic approaches for dealing with behaviours rather than categories of feelings, such as 'depression' and 'despair'. For example: 'When you are depressed how does that show? What do you do with yourself? What effect does this have on your relationships with other people? What would be different in your life if you did not feel like that? What might you do that is different?' This is also a useful approach to use for patients who express extreme anxiety, to the extent that they feel that their symptoms will become overwhelming. For example: 'You say that you'll "crack-up" if this carries on, what do you mean by "crack-up"? What will happen to you? Will you cry, scream, lie on the floor, vomit, stop eating? How long do you think that would go on for?' The therapeutic effect is that 'madness' is to some extent demystified by breaking it down into behaviours. The counsellor also 'floods' the patient with ideas about what happens in madness, which may reduce the potency of the patient's thoughts and make the manifestations potentially less threatening.

The counsellor may feel unclear about how to proceed from the point where

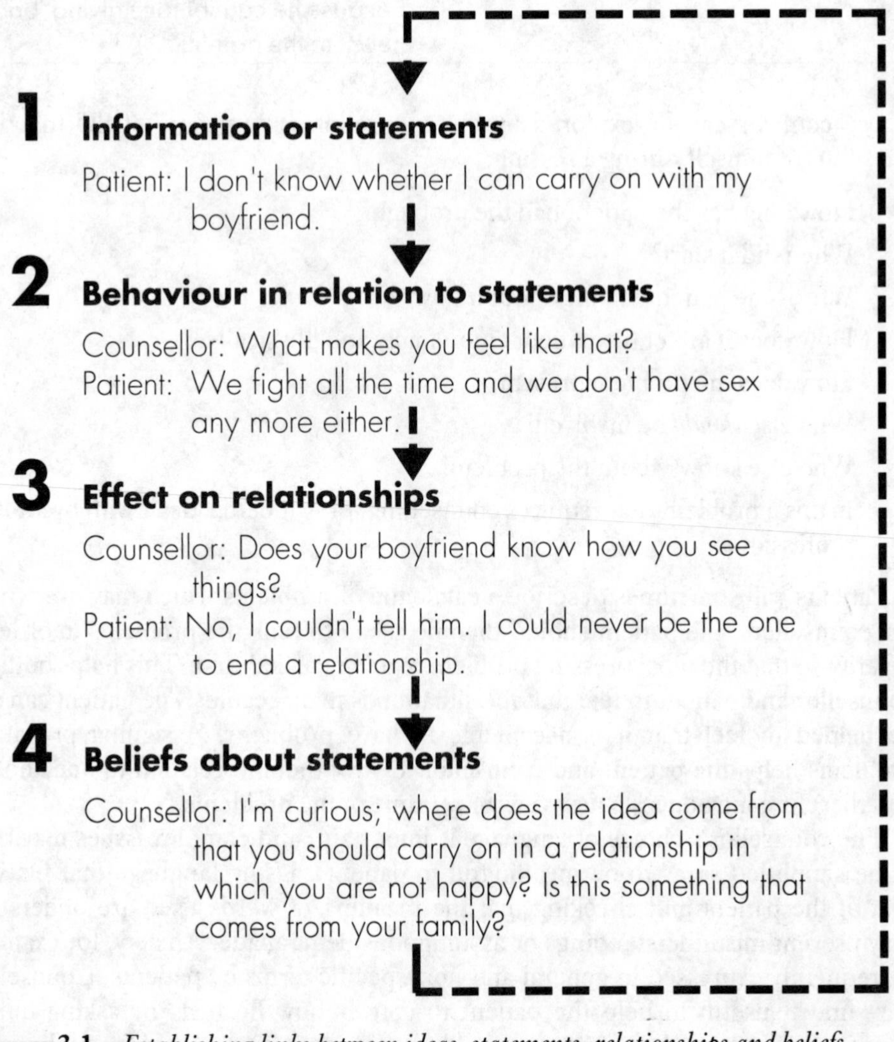

1 Information or statements

Patient: I don't know whether I can carry on with my boyfriend.

2 Behaviour in relation to statements

Counsellor: What makes you feel like that?
Patient: We fight all the time and we don't have sex any more either.

3 Effect on relationships

Counsellor: Does your boyfriend know how you see things?
Patient: No, I couldn't tell him. I could never be the one to end a relationship.

4 Beliefs about statements

Counsellor: I'm curious; where does the idea come from that you should carry on in a relationship in which you are not happy? Is this something that comes from your family?

Figure 3.1 *Establishing links between ideas, statements, relationships and beliefs.*

some behavioural description of the problem has been provided. Sometimes the lead which the counsellor should follow is not immediately evident after the counsellor has a description of the patient's behaviour in relation to a problem. The process is made easier if the counsellor tries to establish links between ideas or statements, behaviours, relationships and beliefs. Figure 3.1 illustrates how this can be done.

Patients seeking help usually want to feel they are being understood by professionals who counsel them. There are several ways of showing this. The counsellor may nod from time to time or reflect on what has been said. A strong confirmation to the patient that he is being heard is to use the patient's own words to form the next question. For example, if a patient were to say: 'I am concerned that my closest friend does not know that I have HIV', the counsellor may then say: 'What concerns you the most about your friend knowing that you have HIV?'. We use the following framework for therapeutically exploring the problem:

Show empathy:	Respect the patient's views and ideas. Use the patient's language.
Validate:	Use co-operative and non-confronting language.
Amplify:	Talk more about the problem and take care not to digress from it until the particular problem is either solved or a new problem becomes more pressing.
Add complexity:	Ask questions of the patient. If an idea or problem seems simple or obvious, become curious and add complexity to the idea. The answers to questions should lead to further questions.
Simplify:	Complex ideas should be simplified.
Reframe:	Give new meaning to ideas and problems.
Understand slowly:	Do not jump to conclusions. Do not make assumptions.

WHAT IS THE PROBLEM?

The counsellor need not presume either the presence or the nature of a problem until it is defined or confirmed by the patient or a system of which he is a part. These systems may include his own personal and social milieu, the professional health and social care systems, or the wider social and political system. An example of how social and political pressures may lead to the creation of a problem is the effect on the general population of the UK Government Health Education Programme. Until the beginning of the programme in 1986, HIV was not seen as a major health problem in the general population. This was despite the fact that over 500 cases of AIDS had already been diagnosed. The health education campaign led to serious strains on parts of the health service when large numbers of people sought advice and HIV testing. HIV had suddenly been defined as a social problem of relevance to the wider population.

The definition of the problem may reflect not necessarily only the stage of illness the patient has reached but also the professional background of the counsellor. A doctor, for example, may view HIV as mainly a medical problem, whereas a social worker may focus on the psychological and social implications of illness. Some patients who do not have noticeable clinical symptoms may have the problem of how to keep their HIV status a secret from others. Those who are hospitalized and cared for in an HIV ward may have the problem of explaining their condition to friends and relatives, who may have had suspicions but no confirmation about the patient's illness. A problem may also shift from person to person over time. In the case of one man who had kept his HIV diagnosis a secret from all his family, the problem of dealing with his family was transformed to the health care staff when the patient died. The family wanted explanations about why his body was labelled as 'infected' with a 'biohazard' warning. They wanted to know why his body was put into a bag and why they could not view it. This resulted in the staff having to deal with the problem of providing an explanation without breaching confidentiality.

The way in which patients view HIV as a problem will in part be a response to how others view it. A gay man may find that the stigma attached to homosexuality is a greater problem. In other words, there may be times when the social aspect overrides the medical implications. There is a reciprocal and circular relationship between the problem and its context. One or both may change at any moment in relation to the other. The problem therefore may change from session to session and over time. In a field in which there are rapid advances, the counsellor needs to be flexible in his working practice so as to accommodate to changes in many parts of the system. In one session the counsellor may be discussing safer sex practices with a couple, one of whom is HIV-positive. At the next session, they may be talking about the possibility of a drug trial. The following case example illustrates how a problem about HIV highlights a wider problem in a marriage.

CASE EXAMPLE A: Fear of Aids as a distance regulator in a marriage

Mr C. made an appointment to see an HIV counsellor as he was worried that he might have contracted HIV. At the initial counselling session it emerged that he was married with two children, aged 24 and 21. He had had two sexual encounters with other men over the past three years. His view was that no one in the family was aware he was bisexual.

They discussed in the session what it would mean for him if he were HIV-positive, if his wife and children were to find out that he was bisexual, and the implications for all of them if he were to become unwell. Mr C. stated towards the end of the session that his marriage had not been good for at least five years and that the situation had deteriorated since his children had left home. He had started to use work as an excuse for coming home late. It was hypothesized that the children's leaving home had aggravated an unsettled marriage. He had found some sexual enjoyment outside the marriage as a means of revitalizing himself. A recent media campaign, coupled with his own guilt, had forced him to make a decision about his marriage. The threat of HIV and coming for the test was the point of the crisis.

The counsellor was able to explore how an HIV test result might influence his decision about the marriage. Mr C. decided to have the test. He had been protecting his wife from possible infection by not having a sexual relationship with her for the last two years and he agreed not to change this until there could be some assessment of his HIV status. He was found to be HIV-negative and arrangements were made for him to have a follow-up test three months later in order to confirm the result, as there was some suggestion that he might recently have had a risky sexual encounter. After the result was given to him, Mr C. said that he was relieved, but that a new problem had arisen. He felt he would have to make a decision about his relationship with his wife but that he had a dilemma. On the one hand he wanted to leave his wife and perhaps pursue a relationship with another man whom he had recently met. On the other hand, he was very concerned about the social stigma of being bisexual or homosexual and about his increased risk for HIV. The counsellor suggested that the patient might want to bring his wife to a joint session. Mr C. seemed relieved and he readily agreed. He said that he would think of a way of suggesting a joint meeting together with his wife and the counsellor.

WITH WHOSE PROBLEM IS THE COUNSELLOR DEALING?

The patient is but one part of the system with which the counsellor works. Invariably there are other systems, including members of the health care team and the support network of the patient. Each of these groups or individuals may have a different view of the problem, and each has its own validity. An HIV-infected asymptomatic patient may, for example, be referred by a nurse in an out-patient department who is concerned about the patient as he keeps checking his body for signs of skin problems and, in particular, for Kaposi's sarcoma. In addressing the presenting problem one task for the counsellor is to consider and discuss the nurse's concerns and beliefs about the patient and his 'obsessional' behaviour.

The immediate task is to obtain a definition of the specific problem and try to identify for whom this is a problem. The patient's lover, a member of his family or someone in the health care team could all be affected. The redefinition of the problem can start at the beginning of the session by exploring different people's views. The following case example illustrates how the focus of the problem in counselling shifted to different family members at different stages of care and bereavement counselling:

CASE EXAMPLE B: Depression

This example illustrates the importance of defining the problem. Changing the referrer's view of the problem made it possible to work with the counsellor towards its resolution. Andrew, aged 21, was first found to be HIV-antibody-positive in an out-patient dermatology clinic. He had recently left home and come to live in London away from his parents. Andrew's relationship with his parents had been tense for about 18 months, as his parents had suspected that he was gay, but this had not been openly discussed in the family. His move to London was an attempt to become more independent of his parents and to lead a more open life. When Andrew first visited the skin clinic he was worried about a 'blotch' on his face which was later diagnosed as Kaposi's sarcoma. He felt like a marked person, estranged from his family, anxious about how his friends might react and unable to meet new people and start relationships. A doctor in the clinic referred Andrew to an HIV counsellor. In the concluding paragraph of the referral note, the doctor stated: 'The patient would probably benefit from individual counselling in order to help him to come to terms with his illness. I feel that this is the key to his depression.'

The doctor was invited to the first session and it was agreed that the counsellor would interview the patient but he would consult with the doctor from time to time in the session.

A considerable amount of the session was used to explore the possible effects of Andrew's homosexuality and illness on the family. The counsellor and doctor had agreed in the pre-session discussion that Andrew might have difficulties in sharing the diagnosis with friends and family. Andrew and the counsellor rehearsed a conversation that he might have with his parents. He was anxious that his parents might interfere with the way he had chosen to live and use his illness as a means to get him to come home and treat him as a child again. Andrew was very concerned that his parents and particularly his younger brother, who was 16, 'would be shattered' if they heard that he was seriously ill, but he did not feel he could hide it from them indefinitely. The younger brother had been seen at a child guidance clinic for a year for disruptive behaviour at school.

In the post-session discussion, the doctor expressed the thought that Andrew seemed more anxious than depressed. The anxiety stemmed from Andrew's dilemma of wanting to tell his family about the HIV diagnosis but fearing the impact of this and its potential to take away his new-found freedom. It was the doctor's suggestion, at the end of the session, that Andrew might want to bring his parents and brother to the next or any other session if he wanted.

Andrew telephoned before the next session to say that the family would be coming. Two family sessions were held over the following ten weeks. In that time, themes relating to social stigma, fear of contamination, parental guilt and issues surrounding death in the family were discussed. At the end of the third session Andrew's mother stated that his brother had been doing much better at school recently and that, for the time being, she did not feel that the family sessions were needed. The others, including the doctor, agreed. The hypothesis was that the secret surrounding Andrew's sexual orientation and illness had been dealt with and that Andrew had shown that he was able to live on his own in London. He was no longer depressed, in the doctor's opinion.

Two individual meetings were held with Andrew and the counsellor over the next six months. Andrew died suddenly from an infection a year after his initial diagnosis. His parents subsequently made contact with the counsellor, requesting a session in order to talk about their loss.

WHEN THE APPARENT SOLUTION BECOMES PART OF THE PROBLEM

It is important to examine other sources of problems in counselling. In some cases, the referring person may create a new view of the problem in the light of his professional opinion, which may even exacerbate the problem. For any problem to exist, it must first be defined by someone as a problem and this definition must be accepted by at least one other person (Maturana *et al.*, 1988). In a counsellor's conversations with a patient, he has the opportunity to confirm or refute problems. This is illustrated by two statements of professional opinion: 'From what I have heard, I do not think there is anything seriously wrong with you and I'm not sure there is any need for further meetings', which conveys an entirely different message from 'This seems a very serious problem and we should meet on a regular basis for several months.'

A professional makes explicit or implies something about the *nature* of the problem when he makes a referral. The referrer may, for example, mention that the patient is 'depressed'. At the same time, a view is conveyed about the person *for whom* this is a problem, be it the patient, a family member or a member of the health care team. The referrer also indicates *what should be done* about the problem. If the referrer, for example, suggests that the patient sees a psychiatrist, the message may be conveyed that there is an organic or biochemical basis to the behaviour, whereas if the referral were made to a psychotherapist, there might be a belief that there were problems in the early development of that person or anxiety about the illness. No referral is therefore a completely neutral gesture. Some consensus about the problem between referrers and counsellors is needed in order to ensure that patients are satisfactorily managed. The case example below illustrates how lack of consensus was a problem with a patient in a clinic and how similar problems can be resolved.

CASE EXAMPLE C: The attempted solution becomes a problem

Gregory, a 44-year-old man with advanced HIV disease, was regularly seen by a physician in a medical out-patient unit. He had been successfully treated for *Pneumocystis carinii* pneumonia on two previous occasions, but was beginning to become unwell again. The counsellor had been seeing the patient every three months to review how he was coping with his diagnosis, treatment and relationships with others.

At his most recent counselling session, Gregory walked in, sat down and said to the counsellor: 'Dr Stephens says I should see a psychiatrist'. Apparently, Gregory had described himself to Dr Stephens as being 'paranoid' and 'depressed'. He qualified this with the doctor by saying that he also thought that his being moody was a natural response to his illness. Gregory disagreed with the physician's view that he should see a psychiatrist. He said that he had financial and physical constraints which put limitations on his life and prevented him from going out as much as he would like to. Having to go to a psychiatrist would, in his opinion, change his view about himself: 'I would be a real nutcase'. He did not have that view of himself in that meeting. Additionally, he stated that it would make his everyday problems seem all the more complex.

This situation presented the counsellor with a dilemma. On the one hand, the counsellor agreed that some of the patient's depressed behaviour was probably a consequence both of his being ill and of his social problems. On the other hand, the patient agreed that he was depressed but did not want to take up a referral to a psychiatrist as he believed that this would compound his problems.

This case illustrates that it can be helpful to ask patients how they think some of their problems might best be solved before offering what may seem the right or best solution. There are several options for the counsellor in the above example. The counsellor might agree with the view of the doctor and suggest that it is a good idea for the patient to consult a psychiatrist. There might then be several levels to the psychosocial management of the patient. These might include the input of a psychiatrist, a counsellor and others all working with the same patient. A second option might be for the counsellor to agree that the patient should see the psychiatrist but to decide to hold off counselling sessions until such time as the sessions with the psychiatrist come to an end. A third option could be to disagree with the doctor about the need for a referral to a psychiatrist. This might put the counsellor in conflict with his medical colleagues, which could also have serious consequences for the patient.

The counsellor might ask the doctor: 'Having spoken to Gregory today, there seem to be some issues that we need to discuss. How do you think the patient's psychological problems should best be managed? If the patient were to see a psychiatrist, how do you think this might affect his view of himself? What new problems do you see arising from having a psychiatrist involved in this case? What advantages might there be? How do you see the work of a counsellor in relation to that of a psychiatrist with such a patient?' By asking questions such as these, it is possible to begin to examine the options open to the professionals and their potential consequences.

The counsellor may feel that the patient is coping despite his unhappiness. The referrer may want the patient attended to by someone else in his busy clinic and suggest the patient sees a psychiatrist in order to pass on the responsibility for assessing and managing the patient's anxiety and depression. On the other hand, the patient may express feelings of unhappiness, but be content not to do anything significantly to change this. The psychiatrist in turn may be faced with a 'resistant' patient rather than one who is 'paranoid' or 'depressed'. It may be that a lack of consensus over the nature of problems and how they should be dealt with can lead to unforeseen difficulties in the management of a patient. These differences between professionals must be resolved first.

PROBLEMS ARISING FROM NOT PROPERLY DEFINING PROBLEMS

Lack of concurrence over the definition of a patient's problem, and indeed over the purpose of referring a patient for counselling, can lead to additional problems for the counsellor, the patient and the referring person. In our experience, additional problems have included: the patient not keeping appointments; the patient resisting counselling; the patient's problem becoming worse than it already is; conflict between the referrer and counsellor; and referrals being made at a time when very little counselling can be done.

Whenever problems similar to these arise in the course of counselling, the counsellor should look beyond the counsellor–patient interaction to the wider system for some understanding of what is happening. He may also look to the wider caring system, including the family, health care team and the hospital system. Much of our work has involved meeting with our referrers in order to discuss views of the purpose and goals of HIV counselling and the range of referrals that might be appropriate (Bor, Miller and Perry, 1988).

PROBLEMS IN COUNSELLING RELATING TO THE COMPETENCE OF THE COUNSELLOR

The practice of skilled professional psychotherapy and counselling requires many years of supervised training and experience. All therapists or counsellors are expected to seek supervision or to refer cases which are beyond their competence, irrespective of their level of experience. Wherever possible, counsellors should arrange for regular supervision. This can make counsellors feel supported in their work and able to grow professionally: two often-overlooked ingredients of good working practice. In some cases, barriers from within the counsellor may stand in the way of progress in the course of counselling a patient. These may stem from underdeveloped theoretical ideas and a lack of therapeutic skills. A personal difficulty with particular issues or processes in counselling can impede the resolution of problems. A drive or mission to make people feel better, for example, may result in repetitive cycles of 'emotional first aid' which may not help a patient in dealing with his concerns about dying.

Where the counsellor feels that the problem has become too difficult to deal with, there is a danger that he may become 'infected' with the same emotional problems as those of the patient unless more experienced help is sought. A number of issues may contribute to this: the patient's loneliness and isolation resulting from the social stigma associated with HIV; his fear of the unknown and uncertainty; and the counsellor's inability to take away all of the patient's emotional pain. Most counsellors are responsive to feelings of competence which are challenged when the counsellor is required or expected to provide a solution to a problem which he may be unable to solve. A patient may, for example, convey to a counsellor that he has become increasingly suicidal. Under these conditions, the counsellor should discuss with the patient the need for a referral to a psychiatrist or request the patient's permission for an experienced supervisor to join their session to help make an assessment of the patient's mental state.

CONCLUSION

The counsellor's task in exploring the patient's problems includes providing the physical and emotional setting and information which help patients to make their own decisions. The patient may be helped to make decisions and to sustain emotional growth even in the face of potential medical and psychosocial problems. In order to achieve this, counsellors need to keep up to date with developments in the field of HIV disease. They need not assume responsibility for making important decisions for patients. Patients can be helped to examine difficulties before they become major problems, placing counselling in the domain of preventive medicine.

By enabling patients to clarify their concerns, it is possible to begin to reframe them by asking questions which seek to place problems in a relational context. Effective counselling depends on a clear definition of the problem. This guides the counsellor in his task and helps to determine when the problem has been solved or become manageable. There is a dynamic and interactive relationship between the questions asked, the therapeutic interventions and the tasks in counselling. We describe some further tasks in systemic HIV counselling in the next chapter.

FOUR

Tasks in Systemic HIV Counselling

Some therapists believe that they have a better sense of reality than their clients. I think it's much more clear and simple for the therapist to give that up and just say, 'I'm curious about the reality that the family created.'

Gianfranco Cecchin

INTRODUCTION

Many patients seek counselling because they feel they have become 'stuck'. In this instance the task of the counsellor is to co-create with the patient new beliefs and ideas about a situation or problem that will enable the patient and his family to adapt to changes brought about by illness. There are several counselling tasks that guide the counsellor in leading the session. The goal is to determine whether there are any problems, to discuss the context of problems and to explore ideas about how illness in general, and HIV in particular, may affect people's beliefs and relationships.

This chapter presents a summary of the theoretical ideas discussed in the preceding chapters as well as some additional counselling tasks, and places them in their clinical context. Examples are provided in order to clarify the tasks of the counsellor and illustrate how to explore certain issues in the context of HIV counselling sessions. These are not comprehensive case studies, but rather brief vignettes which link a theoretical idea with clinical practice. Some systemic tasks are described below:

Tasks

1 *To create a reality with the patient which fits with the patient's current world view and which will sustain him through periods of change which lie ahead.* EXAMPLE:

In the case of a married man with advanced HIV disease, one reality may be how he sees his role as a husband and a father and how this will continue in view of his medical diagnosis, both while he is alive and after his death. Questions which may need consideration include: How will he continue in his role? Who else might take on some of the role? What does he want to preserve?

2 *To elicit all of the problems, as the patient sees them, and then to decide in which relationship areas he needs to work first; that is, to assign priorities to problems for resolution.* EXAMPLE:

A bisexual, married HIV-infected man with children and a boyfriend may want to decide with whom he must first make peace. He may have to consider for whom the problem is the most urgent or distressing. Furthermore, he will need to identify which aspects of the problem require solutions, including sex, the future of relationships, his relationships in the context of other relationships, infectivity and the maintenance of relationships. In so doing, a new set of values and beliefs will emerge in his life and relationships.

3 *To determine whether any part, or which part, of the caring system has defined a problem and to have a conversation about the problem.* EXAMPLE:

A patient came to a counsellor and stated: 'Dr Jones says I must see a counsellor because I have HIV. But I don't have mental problems.' The counsellor responded by saying: 'What do you think it was that made Dr Jones refer you?' 'I did say to him that I was having problems with my husband', replied the patient.

4 *To bring forth in understandable language the problem that is described and co-create, with the counsellor, the reality of the problem.* EXAMPLE:

Patient:	I am depressed; having HIV is getting me down.
Counsellor:	Who else notices you are depressed?
Patient:	No one.
Counsellor:	When you are depressed, how would other people recognize you are depressed?
Patient:	I go out less.
Counsellor:	Who would you most like to notice?
Patient:	My wife.
Counsellor:	What difficulty might you have in showing her you are depressed?
Patient:	Well, she says I should look on the bright side and shouldn't get myself down because that will make me ill.
Counsellor:	Does she ever get depressed?
Patient:	Often.
Counsellor:	What would happen if you were both depressed at the same time?
Patient:	It would be unbearable. We wouldn't be able to 'jump-start' each other to get out of it.

5 *To retain a degree of neutrality in relation to decisions patients make throughout the counselling process.* EXAMPLE:

Patient: I'm not going to tell my wife that I have come for an HIV test.
Counsellor: If you were to tell her, how might she react?
Patient: She would want to leave me.
Counsellor: What might be some of the advantages and disadvantages of your being on your own?

6 *To help the patient to continue to grow and develop.* EXAMPLE:

A young, HIV-infected woman attends for counselling.
Counsellor: If I were to ask you what the most important implication is for you on hearing your test result, what might you say?
Patient: Well, what is the point of going to university?
Counsellor: How might it be for you, say, if ten years from now, looking back, you had decided to go or not to go to university?
Patient: Maybe I won't be here in ten years to look back.
Counsellor: How much future do you think you need to plan for?
Patient: I really have no idea. Everything seems in such a muddle.
Counsellor: What is more important for you right now: the present or the future?

7 *To replace the responsibility for problem-solving with those who define the problem.* EXAMPLE:

Patient: Tell me, who should I tell first about my diagnosis: my mother or my lover?
Counsellor: What is most difficult for you about making this decision?
Patient: That they don't even know I'm using drugs.
Counsellor: How might you tell them?
Patient: I don't know.
Counsellor: Let's think about your mother first. How might you begin to tell her?

8 *To examine with the patient the problem as it is defined and its implications for other relationships.* EXAMPLE:

Patient: I'm not interested in using condoms. How will I ever get a girlfriend if I can't screw around like my mates?
Counsellor: Aside from sex, what else have you got going for you? So, you have sex, then what?
Patient: It's not really like me to screw around. But it's the pressure, you see. It's my mates. They'll think I'm bent if I'm not like them.

Counsellor:	Do any of them use condoms?
Patient:	I doubt it.
Counsellor:	If one of your girlfriends became infected, then . . . .
Patient:	Then she'd have to stick with me.
Counsellor:	Is that the only way you can see yourself having a permanent relationship?
Patient:	Sometimes.
Counsellor:	Chris, I can't make you protect your sexual partners, just as I can't make a girl want to be your lover. But I'm also not sure that you're looking very far into the future. How strong can a relationship become if it starts out with such big secrets?

9 *To help the patient system not to become stuck around problems and to help a psychologically vulnerable person to cope with additional stresses and thereby possibly prevent the development of major psychological problems. This may engender addressing fears of death and dying.* EXAMPLE:

A patient lapsed into what seemed to be a depression on being told she had HIV. She stopped work, ended her contact with her family, failed to keep appointments with her doctor, stayed indoors most of the time and raised considerable anxiety among the doctors and nurses caring for her. Through counselling, she was able to discuss some of her worries about her health and social relationships. She decided to resume medical appointments and some of her physical problems were attended to. In time, with the improvement in her health, she decided to resume part-time work. Through further counselling, she made plans about her future, moved into a new flat and initiated social contact with her family.

10 *To talk about the concept of unpredictability with the patient, which is reality for him. The patient's concern about unpredictability may be reflected in questions such as: 'Why should I carry on?', 'How should I carry on?', 'How will the disease progress?' and 'What should I do differently?'* EXAMPLE:

Patient:	What will happen to me next?
Counsellor:	What worries you most about what will happen next?
Patient:	Maybe that I'd die and there are many things that I still want to do.
Counsellor:	What would be most left undone if you were to die suddenly, for whatever reason?
Patient:	That I haven't made a will and my children are so young . . . .
Counsellor:	If you didn't have HIV, would there be anything to prevent you from making a will? Perhaps everyone should have one. There are accidents and unexpected events in all of our lives.
Patient:	I suppose you're right. Look at all the recent rail and air disasters.

11 *To view HIV as the entrée to other problems, such as relationship difficulties. HIV, in this context, is also a symptom of other problems and need not necessarily be the main problem or the enduring problem.* EXAMPLE:

A patient who persistently worries whether he is infected with HIV may come to understand that his worry interferes with his ability to enter into new relationships.

12 *To examine the difficulties that arise from the patient's apparent wish for some isolation to avoid social stigma and transmission of HIV, in contrast with a desire to be more involved with the family, a common feeling in people living with a life-threatening condition.* EXAMPLE:

Counsellor: You say that you have not felt like having relationships. Can you say a little more about that?
Patient: What's the point in starting a relationship if it has to end?
Counsellor: Do you feel that about all relationships?
Patient: I suppose not all. I see you. I see my father. I've got to know new people in the hospital. But that's not the same as a sexual relationship.
Counsellor: So you have started some new relationships. At what stage in a new sexual relationship would you talk about HIV or the general risks in sex?
Patient: Not until I was comfortable with the person and I trusted them a bit.
Counsellor: So what seems most difficult; meeting people, starting a relationship or keeping a relationship?
Patient: Keeping a relationship. I've always had that problem. That's maybe why I've slept around so much in the past. I am terrified of being alone and just as frightened of getting too close.

13 *To help the patient to find a new view of what it means to have HIV.* EXAMPLE:

Counsellor: This may sound a strange question, but has anything good come of your having this diagnosis?
Patient: Yes. It's brought me much closer to my family than I was before.

14 *To normalize the views, feelings and experience of the patient.* EXAMPLE:

Patient: I feel so alone and I don't want to talk to people about having this . . . well, this problem of HIV.
Counsellor: I would be surprised if at some stage you didn't feel like that. When do you think it will feel different for you?

15 *To help the patient to engage with his natural support system (family, friends, and others), if this is what he desires, and at the same time to prevent health care staff who feel compelled to 'mother' patients from crossing professional boundaries. Failure to address this can lead to feelings of burnout in staff. Supervision can help counsellors to recognize these boundaries, thereby increasing their professional competence.* EXAMPLE:

Patient:	It feels so good when I come for counselling. I feel safe and I don't have any big pressures.
Counsellor:	Apart from our sessions, where else do you feel supported and safe?
Patient:	With a few good friends, but we don't talk about my illness.
Counsellor:	To whom do you feel closest in the world?
Patient:	My aunt. But I could never tell her about HIV.
Counsellor:	If you were to tell her, do you think that the two of you would get closer or further apart?
Patient:	Much closer. Maybe I wouldn't need to come here so much.
Counsellor:	What do you feel you gain and what do you feel you lose by only telling me how things are for you?

16 *To help patients feel that they have choices. As a consequence of both having a potentially life-threatening condition and being involved with many other health care workers with different views and beliefs, patients may feel that choices are being taken away from them. By reducing choices, one simultaneously takes away a sense of autonomy. In making decisions for patients, such as how to live and die, the counsellor could either make their problems seem worse or create apparent resistance.* EXAMPLE:

Patient:	The doctors tell me that the lymphoma is not responding to treatment.
Counsellor:	What else did they say?
Patient:	Nothing really. I know I'm going to die soon now.
Counsellor:	If you were given the choice to die in hospital or at home, where would you want to be?
Patient:	At home. I want to be able to look at the garden and have the dogs around.
Counsellor:	There are many other things I think we should talk about now. But first, would you like me to arrange for our Home Care and Support Team to visit you?
Patient:	Yes.

CONCLUSION

Whether counselling someone infected with HIV or a person worried about becoming infected, a context for a meaningful conversation can be provided. HIV disease can put severe strains on relationships as people face significant choices. Throughout our lives, we are confronted with numerous difficult communicative situations, and the process of communicating with a person who is unwell or who is known to be dying may be the most difficult of all (Welch-Cline, 1988). The barriers to effective communication affect not only the person with HIV disease, but also the family, partner, friends and health care providers, each of whom may be uncertain about what to say to the other. The counselling tasks described in this chapter consolidate a number of possible leads that counsellors can follow in order to identify and resolve patients' problems.

The complexity and unpredictability of the disease process do not always allow for permanent solutions to be provided. Therefore, the counsellor may attempt, wherever possible, to introduce and create alternative views of the problem which will result in emotional relief. It is important to communicate to a patient that the care-giving team will be there to support him throughout the course of his illness. Using a systemic approach, the tasks of the counsellor will *inter alia* be to bring forth and define the problem and to become aware of the subsystems to be addressed in attempting to resolve the problems. In the context of HIV disease, certain themes appear to recur, for example, secrecy, complexity, difficulties in relationships and interaction, and uncertainty. It is probable that at some stage in the counselling process counsellors will deal with one, some or all of these as they help the patient and others to find an alternative view of the problem and to generate new solutions. The challenging task of either having to give bad news to a patient or helping him to cope with his fear of it is described in the following chapter.

HAROLD BRIDGES LIBRARY
S. MARTIN'S COLLEGE
LANCASTER

FIVE

Preparing Patients for Bad News

Time present and time past are both perhaps present in time future,
and time future constrained in time past.

T.S. Eliot

INTRODUCTION

HIV infection is a medical problem that has focused attention on communicating with patients about their condition; imparting bad news may inevitably be part of this (Hoy, 1985). The problems associated with giving bad news in HIV, and the potential difficulties and barriers this can create in the doctor–patient relationship, are not new to medicine (Buckman, 1984). Most doctors, nurses and other health care providers have considerable experience in this difficult task, although the emphasis on working with young and well-informed patients may be new for some. Difficulty with giving bad news is compounded by the challenge of helping patients diagnosed with HIV infection to manage their concerns and fears about what may happen to them in the future. This may entail addressing issues such as a deterioration in health and the potential for disfigurement, pain, loss, stigma and death.

In this chapter, we examine what may be considered bad news in HIV disease, and what may inhibit health care providers from communicating openly and effectively with patients about their condition. Some guidelines are offered for how to prepare patients for the changes that may lie ahead, to cope with the fears they may have for these changes, and how to give bad news, should the need arise.

THEORETICAL BACKGROUND

The meaning of 'bad news'?

Conventionally the concept of bad news pertains to situations where there is either a feeling of no hope, a threat to an individual's mental or physical well-being, a risk of upsetting an established lifestyle, or where a message is given which conveys to the individual fewer choices in his life. It may be tempting to assume whether news is *good* or *bad* for an individual. News, of whatever kind, is information, whereas the idea that it is either *good* or *bad* is a belief, value judgement or affective response from either the provider or the receiver of the information in a given context.

There are many situations in which health care providers might preface giving news with 'I am sorry to tell you that . . .' or 'I am pleased to tell you . . .', illustrating how value and meaning are attached to information from the outset. Such preconceptions about what is *good* or *bad* news associated with HIV may influence or constrain the patient's range of responses to the information. A patient who is given so-called good news in the form of a negative HIV test by a relieved doctor may feel ashamed to cry or to discuss new problems for himself. For that patient, for example, there may be an element of bad news, as he then feels that there are no excuses for failing in a sexual relationship, whereas his fear of HIV had previously protected him from meeting new partners. Similarly, a patient who feels some relief and more settled in his mind about an AIDS diagnosis may be concerned that the doctor will misconstrue this as denial, emotional blunting or suggestive of a psychiatric disorder (McGuire and Faulkner, 1988).

Clinical experience highlights the value of waiting until the patient attaches meaning to the information before defining it as either good or bad news. This does not mean that health care providers are unaffected by the patient's feelings and responses, but that they should neither make assumptions as to what these may be nor inhibit the patient's spontaneous reactions.

What aspects of bad news do patients with HIV fear?

Those people who have decided to be tested for HIV may be fearful of receiving a positive result. The next fear may be of developing symptoms and having an AIDS-defining illness, such as *Pneumocystis carinii* pneumonia. Bad news for those patients attending for regular monitoring may be a falling CD4 count, or a fear that resistance has developed to a drug being used to treat them where there is no substitute or alternative treatment. A fear of having Kaposi's sarcoma or extreme weight loss, which many patients regard as being obvious or tell-tale signs of HIV disease, features prominently in patients. The news that a child is infected or that the infection has been transmitted to a sexual partner can be devastating. Symptoms of HIV-related neurological impairment may be especially frightening to patients as this may be equated with loss of self-control and 'madness'. Our clinical experience has shown that most patients with HIV have some of the fears that are listed in Table 5.1.

Table 5.1   Patients' main fears

Living with uncertainty.
Disfigurement and pain in the course of illness.
The loss of friends, lovers and the family.
Social stigma from disclosure of relationships, sexual orientation or HIV risk-associated behaviour.
Neurological impairment and the loss of the ability to make decisions for oneself.

Life-sustaining measures, such as mechanical ventilation and resuscitation.
Death and dying.
Making decisions about having children, in some cases.
Unemployment and financial loss.
Loss of a sense of future.
Lack of control and increasing dependence on others.

There are many situations in which bad news may have to be given to patients where there is chronic illness, with the possibility of acute illness superimposed. The range of HIV-related medical conditions is extensive and it is not within the scope of this book to describe all of them. Any condition can give rise to anxiety and distress, and for this reason psychological morbidity may be associated both with a fear of a medical condition or infection, and with having to cope with it.

Patients' psychological responses to a fear of these conditions are mediated by a number of factors. In the case of Kaposi's sarcoma, for example, patients may respond differently, depending on the location, size or contour of the lesion (Harrison, 1988). Social and cultural factors may determine the extent to which patients are distressed by their changing physical appearance. Actors, models and others who depend on their physical appearance may exhibit greater anxiety in relation to the effect of their condition on their work, for example. We have found that some patients find that psychological problems become more pressing after they have been discharged from hospital to convalesce. It seems that the hospital itself may provide a protective social environment for patients. Similarly, the signs and symptoms of neurological disease can impair patients' functions in a number of ways and therefore have different implications for them. These range from apathy, social withdrawal, impaired handwriting, and headaches to memory loss, seizures, dysphasia, hemiparesis and even coma (Elder and Sever, 1988).

What may inhibit health care providers from giving bad news?

In the case of HIV disease there are a number of factors that might make it difficult for health care providers to give bad news to their patients. The majority of patients with HIV are young and an implication of the diagnosis is that they are being told that they may have a shortened life span. Counsellors may witness the erosion of the patient's self-confidence and hopes for the future, and fear being blamed for this. HIV disease requires discussion about sensitive topics with patients, including sex and sexuality, procreation, and ill health. Some health care providers may lack confidence in their counselling skills to discuss these subjects openly and effectively with patients. They may be concerned that they will distress patients if they either tell them the bad news or talk to them about any fears they may have in relation to it. This may stem from a myth that to do so is to tempt fate or to destroy any remaining feelings of hope the patient may have.

Uncertainty about how to respond to the reactions of certain patients who become very emotional, angry or display no feelings may also be unnerving. Some health care providers may be unsure whether their own responses should be personal or professional; to be clinical and aloof, or deeply engaged and possibly also visibly upset together with the patient. They may strongly identify with some patients and their problems, especially if their ages and lifestyles are similar.

Many patients with HIV disease have come to challenge aspects of medical practice and have sought to become more informed and involved in clinical decision-making. This may be unsettling for some professionals who feel more comfortable with the conventional and hierarchically arranged doctor–patient relationship. Not knowing all the answers to questions patients may ask and having insufficient counselling skills may arouse anxiety and tempt some health care providers to delegate the task of communicating to patients about sensitive topics to colleagues. Working alone can also increase stress and tension (McLauchlan, 1990). Giving bad news can lead to time-consuming conversations with patients and this may deter some doctors from being more open with their patients in busy out-patient clinics.

PREPARING PATIENTS FOR BAD NEWS

Unlike accident victims or those with unexpected medical crises, people with HIV disease may in some cases be able to make some practical changes and prepare themselves emotionally for bad news. Talking to patients about their fears for the future is one of the most important therapeutic interventions of a counsellor (Perakyla and Bor, 1991). It provides an opportunity to help patients cope with the anxiety and uncertainty about what may happen to them through the course of their illness. If this is done satisfactorily, the counsellor may even have helped to prevent some psychiatric symptoms in those patients who seem very anxious about addressing their fears. A change for the worse in a patient's clinical condition affects his relationships, his feelings of hope and his view of himself in the context of his illness. For some patients it may mean being open with people about the diagnosis. For patients who are neurologically impaired, an important additional issue may be dealing with a lack of control in relationships. Increasing dependence on others for support and care is one manifestation of this. In addition, this lack of control may be manifested in an inability to interact in relationships in a normal way because of the unpredictability of illness.

Counsellors can see the matter of preparing patients for bad news as an opportunity to open up communication between themselves and the patient by enabling the patient to express his views about care and treatment. Identifying the patient's views can enable him to challenge his beliefs and look at the meaning of bad news from a different perspective. Counsellors are faced with three options regarding the therapeutic management of patients' concerns. These are described below:

Option 1:   Reassure the patient, potentially colluding with denial.

The counsellor can reassure the patient that his fears for the future are probably worse than the reality. This option may be difficult to resist because it can result in an immediate reduction of the patient's anxiety and emotional distress. It is a form of supportive emotional 'first aid' which may be indicated when the patient appears to be isolated and under extreme distress. Given the extent of what is known about HIV disease, however, this reaction is often inappropriate and may serve to 'sweep the fear under the carpet', only to resurface at another point in time. If the counsellor repeatedly reassures the patient, he takes on some of his anxiety and assumes responsibility for some decisions that could be shared. This is more likely to result in feelings of burnout. The counsellor might also be colluding with the patient's denial of the severity of the problem, or potential problem, if false hope is offered.

Option 2:   Impose views on patients when it is too late and possibly face resistance.

A second option is to wait until a crisis occurs before discussing bad news. The patient may be seriously ill with an AIDS-related illness such as *Pneumocystis carinii* pneumonia before his concerns are elicited. This has certain limitations. Patients may be unprepared for bad news; they are not only anxious about their physical condition, but will inevitably have fewer ideas about how they might cope. They may present as anxious, depressed, withdrawn and some will express suicidal thoughts. Psychotherapy is less likely to be successful if the referral and intervention are made when patients are already seriously ill. If referrals for specialist counselling are made at a time of crisis, patients may then seem to be resistant to any intervention by the counsellor. Referrals made when patients are still well tend, on the whole, to have a better outcome.

Option 3:   Use hypothetical and future-orientated questions; avoid denial and resistance.

The third option is to address the potential for bad news and concerns about the future with patients, using hypothetical and future-oriented questions at appropriate times, while patients are still relatively well. The theory behind the use of questions in counselling is described in Chapter 2. There are several advantages to this approach. Patients are still relatively well and they have some distance from potentially serious conditions. If issues are raised and addressed at this stage, patients can plan ahead of crises and they can be helped to view their situation more objectively. The ideas can be put across in a non-confronting way, through the use of questions. It should be noted that denial is sometimes a vital coping strategy for some patients and therefore should not always be viewed as dysfunctional. Patients who indicate that they experience it as too unsettling to talk about their fears for the future should not be pushed to do so. It is unusual to challenge or lay bare a patient's psychological defences in this counselling approach.

Questions can help to make easier the task of dealing with patients' uncertainties.

Counsellors can inoculate patients against extreme stress in the future by having them think about possible problems and how they might cope with them before they actually occur. The main concerns of the patients are thereby addressed and this can also lead to the more efficient use of clinical time. The method emphasizes helping patients to cope on their own, and this may lead to the need for less patient contact. As described in Chapter 2, the patient's hearing the questions asked by the counsellor may be more important than his answers. All questions convey an idea or imply a statement. Questions are a way of giving back to the patient some responsibility for finding solutions to his concerns at a stage when he can realistically be expected to act on them. This use of questions may prevent the staff from becoming overburdened with the patient's needs and worries.

An extract from a case example is described below in order to illustrate the method, its application and effects.

CASE EXAMPLE D: A case of declining health

Jason, a 32-year-old HIV-infected man, was referred to a counsellor by his general practitioner. The doctor was concerned about the patient's current health and he thought that there was a possibility of Jason developing AIDS. The doctor wanted some idea of how the patient might cope if his health deteriorated. The patient had been difficult to assess in the past because he always joked and dismissed questions about how he was managing. The interview began as follows:

Counsellor: Dr James has some concerns about you and he asked me to see you; what do you think he might be concerned about?
In a busy clinic, time is limited and there is a need for counselling to be focused. The main conerns are addressed from the outset.
Patient: The temperatures that don't go away.
Counsellor: What do the temperatures that don't go away mean to you?
It conveys empathy to use the words of the patient to form the next question.
Patient: Maybe that would be the beginning of AIDS . . ..
The counsellor now introduces a hypothetical question as a way of beginning to address 'dreaded issues'. Until now, the counsellor and the doctor have not been able to talk about what might happen if Jason became unwell. The following questions explore who may be available to help Jason and what he might have told them about his condition.
Counsellor: What if the temperatures continue and don't go away; how might you see your situation and how might you cope?
Patient: I would probably want to tell my parents then. If I'm in hospital and I'm too sick to work, I'll give up my job. Until then, I'll keep going as things seem to be all right.
Counsellor: If you reached a stage in your illness when you felt that you could not manage alone, what would you want to do and who would you want to help you?
The answer to this question gives the counsellor some idea about social support and important relationships in the patient's life. The counsellor can also assess the extent to which Jason feels that he wants to share important information with others. The counsellor then returns to the discussion about hypothetical dreaded issues.
Counsellor: Jason, I don't think that we've ever discussed this, but I would be interested to know whether you have thought about what might happen if it came to a stage some time in the future, when crucial decisions had to be made about your care and treatment. I always ask patients if they have

	particular views about how they might wish to be treated if, say, a ventilator was needed to keep them going.
Patient:	That decision is for Mark [his boyfriend] to make. He and I have talked about this once. We both feel that if either of us has neurological problems or we are just wired-up to a machine, there would be no point in carrying on.
Counsellor:	Would anything give you hope in difficult medical situations?
Patient:	Having Mark there to take care of me and to make decisions for me. I guess that as long as people are open and honest, I can trust them. When I trust people, I feel more secure and confident about things.

Providing an opportunity to talk about these concerns at an early stage can help patients to take some control over their care and management. Although it is the medical staff who have ultimate responsibility for clinical decisions, they may be helped in their task if they know the patient's views. Fahrner *et al.* (1987) have reported that a significant proportion of patients with HIV whom they surveyed had firm ideas about how much treatment and care they would find acceptable in these difficult clinical situations. These views should be checked as they may change over time.

GIVING PATIENTS BAD NEWS

Although there is no right or wrong way of conveying bad news, some principles and techniques may help the health care provider to do this with confidence. An example of breaking news to a patient is used to demonstrate some of the principles.

Timing

An assessment of the patient's physical, psychological and social circumstances, the available support resources and the clinician's readiness to discuss the news may determine when bad news is to be given.

Practical details

First attend to some practical details. These include ensuring that there is privacy, a reasonably comfortable room and calm ambience, sufficient time available, and that links have been established with other colleagues who can offer support to the patient afterwards if necessary.

Facilitate communication

Establish rapport and trust with the patient by introducing yourself, defining the purpose of the meeting, maintaining eye contact, and being aware of body postures, such as leaning forward. Convey information without disguising it in language that is either vague or ambiguous. For example:

Doctor: You have been unwell for the last few days and you have what we call *Pneumocystis carinii* pneumonia, which is an AIDS-related lung infection.
Patient: So what does that mean for me?
Doctor: We are treating you for this infection, and there is a good chance of preventing recurrence of the *Pneumocystis* pneumonia, but as you know, we can't completely cure HIV disease.

Check knowledge and information

On hearing bad news many people are unable to absorb anything further and do not hear what is being said. It may be tempting to flood them with information, as hope can be conveyed by discussing the possibilities of current treatments and drug trials. Talking incessantly to a patient immediately after he has been given bad news may reflect the counsellor's need to fill a silence or avoid talking to the patient about his feelings of hopelessness. Rather, the counsellor should check again what the patient has remembered and understood about what he has been told about investigations and laboratory tests. The counsellor should review how much he wants to know about the results of any subsequent tests and investigations.

Maintain some neutrality

Some neutrality can be maintained by responding thoughtfully and professionally to a patient's emotional outburst, by not showing surprise or making value-laden judgements, such as: 'There's no need to be upset; it's not the end of the world.' Neutrality enables patients to respond more freely, without the feeling that they are being judged, or that certain responses are expected of them. For example:

Patient: I can't believe I have AIDS. It's the end. (Patient sobs)
Counsellor: What is the hardest for you to believe right now?
Patient: (Continues to sob loudly)
Counsellor: (Pause, passes patient a box of tissues) What would help you the most right now?
Patient: Nothing. Though I wish I could think straight.
Counsellor: Let's talk about the things that are in your mind.
Patient: I'll be all right in a minute ... (pause) ... this is the day I've feared the most. Actually things look a bit clearer now. How is AIDS different to having HIV?

Show empathy

The counsellor should convey warmth and caring in his manner and discussion with the patient. The way in which the counsellor introduces the topic of bad news will influence to some degree how the patient responds. It is sometimes helpful to embroider a little and use prefaces such as: 'I was wondering whether you had ever thought how things might be if this infection does not clear up as quickly as last time?' Putting oneself 'down' also encourages the patient to talk more freely. For example: 'You may think that some of my questions seem a bit odd, but I can't help wondering whether . . .'. Showing patients that the counsellor is not afraid to discuss their concerns, no matter what these might be, is a way of showing empathy and closely tracking the thoughts of the patient.

Counsellor: You said that AIDS means 'the end'. What would that mean to you?
Patient: It's hard to talk about.
Counsellor: Perhaps you could try.
Patient: Well, what will it be like being dead? I often wonder.
Counsellor: What do you wonder about?
Patient: Whether it's the real end, or just the end of my time on earth.
Counsellor: What would you do differently if it were possible to know whether it was?
Patient: (Smiles)

Enquire about past experiences of bad news

Emphasis should be placed on how patients have coped with personal difficulties in the *past*, and the counsellor should help them to consider how they might cope *now* and in the *future*. This encourages them to consider how they might manage if the news did turn out to be bad for them. Examples of questions are:

Have you ever been given news in the past that made you very frightened and unsure how to respond?

How did you deal with it?

How might this experience help you in what we have been discussing today?

Ask questions about the future

Using future-orientated and hypothetical questions can help patients to think about the implications of bad news, as described above. The counsellor can ask the patient how he sees his future with the new information and what new problems may arise from this. A patient who has developed Kaposi's sarcoma may, for example, be asked some of the following questions in the course of counselling:

When others see these lesions, do you think they are likely to help you more or to withdraw from you?

What will the lesions tell them about you?

How do you see your chances of finding a new lover or partner now that you have Kaposi's?

Have you thought about seeing the consultant who advises patients about cosmetic applications to disguise the lesions?

How might it affect your relationship with the nurses if they see you so upset and there is nothing they feel they can do to help you?

Convey some measure of hope

Information about treatments and uncertainties in medicine may help patients to consider realistically other possible courses or outcomes of their illness. This helps to convey some hope for the future and is illustrated in the following dialogue:

Counsellor: AIDS means that your immune system is not fighting off infections properly. What do you know about the treatments we can offer to help keep some of them away, and to help you right now?

Patient: I've heard about AZT.

Counsellor: Yes, antiviral treatments like AZT may help to make you feel better and to slow down the process of getting ill, but there are other treatments that we can now offer you to try and prevent other infections occurring.

Patient: Does this mean pills for life?

Counsellor: It may mean pills, but not necessarily all the time. Some treatments are not in pill form. It means we need to see you more often to assess what would be best for you.

Identify the patient's support network

Identify who else may be available to offer support to the patient. This helps patients look to their natural support network outside the health care setting, and reduces the dependence on professional staff.

Ending the session

After people have been given bad news, the last few moments of the session are particularly important, as patients' main concerns invariably arise at this point if they have not already been addressed. It is tempting to assume that patients have retained and understood what they have been told. Asking patients to summarize what they remember and to correct any misunderstandings, before the session ends, is a helpful way of checking what they have retained. If this is not done, the patient might leave having heard only the positive or negative aspects of the news, both of which may increase his risk of reactive depression, denial, anxiety and even suicide. It is also important to clarify what additional help the patient may need or be willing to accept, and what he can still do on his own in the light of his changing circumstances. A plan should be made for follow-up contact in order to contain concerns and anxiety until the next session when they can be addressed.

Provide feedback to colleagues

Discussion and consultation with colleagues can make the task of giving bad news easier by increasing professional support and exploring ideas about how to manage difficult situations for the benefit of patients (Speck, 1991). In addition, colleagues involved in the care of the patient should be provided with a summary of what was said in the session with the patient. In this way, any problems that may subsequently arise can be dealt with by other staff. This conveys co-ordinated care.

CASE EXAMPLE E: The meaning of bad news in a relationship

Ideas have been suggested in this chapter for how to give bad news effectively. The therapeutic themes that should be addressed in relation to bad news are: the meaning it has for the patient, his relationships, and his view of the present and future. The case vignette below illustrates how bad news reshuffles a patient's views and understanding of his condition and of his relationship with his partner.

Fred, an HIV-positive man, was infected several years ago through sharing injecting needles. A diagnosis of AIDS was made at his last medical appointment following *Pneumocystis carinii* pneumonia. This was the first time that he had spoken about his diagnosis with the medical team. When Fred was told that he had AIDS he started to cry. The counsellor asked Fred what had upset him. He said he was crying both because of the emotional upset that he had long feared would accompany the diagnosis and the relief that the time of uncertainty of living *in the shadow* of an AIDS diagnosis had come to an end.

After a long session, Fred went home and broke the news to Vince, his boyfriend. Vince was distressed, and it appeared that he had taken the news worse than Fred. They decided that they should both come for a counselling session together. During the session the counsellor explored what the AIDS diagnosis meant for their relationship. Vince felt that this was the beginning of losing his boyfriend, and the beginning of the end of their relationship. The counsellor began to develop an idea during the discussion that Vince might have found it more difficult to receive the news than Fred, and asked the question: 'For whom has the news been hardest?' Their responses confirmed that Fred felt that it was difficult telling his boyfriend that he had had bad news because he feared that Vince would be devastated. This fear was confirmed by Vince's repeated statements that he could see no future for himself without Fred. This in turn compelled Fred to comfort and care for Vince, thus reversing a pattern in their relationship. In the past it was usually Vince who was more demonstrative in his support and care of Fred. The effect of the bad news was that Fred took on a greater caring role in the relationship.

It became clear that bad news in this situation led to a change in the pattern of caring in the relationship. At a later session, Fred expressed concern that looking after Vince had distracted him from thinking about his own future, which he felt was a saviour at the time. It had stopped him from 'cracking up'.

CONCLUSION

Having to give bad news and helping people to cope with it is an important aspect of professional care for people with HIV disease. *How* bad news is given is important and may determine, or at least influence, how the patient subsequently copes and adapts to his changing circumstances.

The approach described in this chapter for counselling patients about difficult issues needs to be used with thought and sensitivity. Asking the patient questions should serve as an invitation to a conversation about difficult issues. An interrogatory interviewing style will not only alienate a patient, but may also be countertherapeutic. The use of hypothetical questions is an approach that requires a high level of training as it focuses on the most painful aspects of living and coping with HIV disease. We feel that it is damaging to patients to ask hypothetical and future-oriented questions that raise their anxiety without addressing what actions they would like to take and how they might cope. In order to retain a sense of balance over feelings of hope and hopelessness about the future, the positive aspects of the patient's coping are always discussed. The counsellor can help to normalize the views of the patient by conveying that these may be uncomfortable conversations to have and difficult decisions to make. It is inappropriate to push patients to talk about their fears for the future when the feedback from them indicates that they are not ready to do this. Addressing patients' concerns about the potential for bad news can help them to feel that they can talk about their worries and show their emotions. Most of the associated worries are probably already in the mind of the patient, and an experienced counsellor will find an appropriate moment to talk to the patient about them.

SIX

Reframing: Creating Balance in Patient Belief Systems

You have to treat death like any other part of life.

Isaac Bashevis Singer

INTRODUCTION

Many psychosocial problems associated with HIV disease are inherently relationship problems. The systemic counselling approach is based on a belief that problems are defined in the context of relationships. From the counsellor's point of view, these problems frequently relate to unpredictability, instability, hopelessness, separateness and their complements. The technique of 'balancing', which is described in this chapter, extends the theory and practice of addressing patients' fears of the future insofar as the technique is the beginning of a counsellor's 'reframe'. Introducing some balance to a patient's belief system is a useful therapeutic intervention for helping him to live with some measure of uncertainty and unpredictability, which is reality for anyone with a potentially life-threatening illness.

The 'balancing' intervention serves to introduce new views and possibilities without falsely reassuring the patient. The approach is firmly embedded in systemic theory and directly reflects the concept of the relativity of people's views and feelings. In Chapter 2, reference was made to Bateson's (1979) idea of difference, which introduces the concept of balance or complementarity. 'Happiness', for example, can only be comprehended in the context of, say, 'unhappiness' or 'despondency'. A range of counselling themes can be discussed with patients in a similar way.

In the course of HIV counselling, a number of themes emerge which can be explored therapeutically by the counsellor with the patient. One of the ideas of systemic counselling is that there are many views of reality. The counsellor can introduce a different view of the problem, that is to reframe the problem. In the words of Campbell and Draper (1985, p. 7), 'Many families who are "stuck" with a problem have lost contact with this recursiveness [multiple views of reality], and the meaning they attach to symptomatic behaviour becomes lineal, that is, "it is bad or it is mad".' One task of the counsellor or therapist in such a case may be to identify beliefs of the patient about his problems and to offer alternate views where appropriate. Thus, it may be useful to address both sides or the complement for a particular theme at different stages of counselling. Some of the most common themes that we have identified in our HIV counselling setting pertaining to patients, presented as complements, are shown in Figure 6.1.

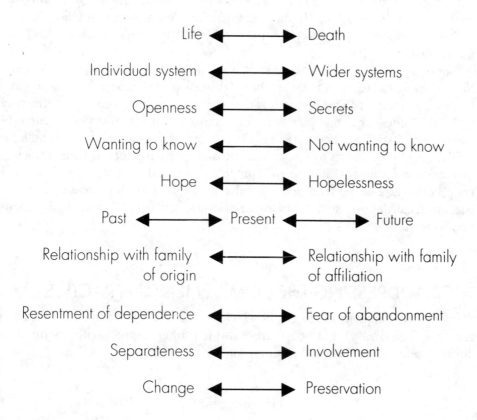

Figure 6.1 *Counselling themes as complements.*

The counsellor may be able to reframe one side of an idea or a problem in the context of the other. Life, for example, may be seen in the context of death and vice versa. The idea of 'balance' is directly related to the theoretical concept of 'difference' (Bateson, 1979), which in turn is associated with the idea of distinctions, which has been previously termed 'cybernetic complementarity' (Keeney, 1983). In most counselling approaches described in the literature about HIV disease, the emphasis is on only one side of the problem, such as death, pathology, loss, depression and dysfunction. By addressing the complement the counsellor may be able to amplify, add complexity to, and ultimately reframe, the patient's view of his problems, as described in Chapter 3. One effect of this may be not only to influence or change the patient's view of his own illness, but it may have a ripple effect on other people's views, such as the family and health care providers.

By conversing with patients through the mode of circular questions (Penn, 1982), new ideas, beliefs and connections may emerge among the patient's family members, friends and even among members of the professional team caring for the patient. In connecting the complementary aspects of an idea, it is hoped that the patient can come to a different understanding of his condition by making new connections in his thinking. In the seemingly hopeless situation of a fatal illness a patient may, for example, recognize the extent of caring and closeness in his family for the first time.

Not trying to change the patient's ideas in any predetermined way may enhance his autonomy and capacity to cope. One of the tasks of the counsellor is to provide a context so that the patient recognizes that *he* is the resource for dealing effectively with difficulties and the potential for confusion that seems to threaten his psychological stability (Parry, 1984). The counsellor can do this, for example, by validating *all* perceptions of the patient and adopting a non-oppositional stance, as may be done through addressing complementary sides of the problem. This counselling task is perhaps much undervalued in a context where there are particularly strong and sometimes even rigid views and beliefs among both patients and professionals.

ADDRESSING THE COMPLEMENT IN PRACTICE

A number of complements or issues which may arise in the course of counselling are described below. Examples are provided where appropriate in order to illustrate how 'balancing' can be initiated in practice.

Life and death

The opportunistic infections associated with a diagnosis of AIDS are often fatal and so the theme of death may be common in conversations with the patient. In order to think about death and its implications for an individual, its complement, life, has to be considered. Thus, it is not possible to think about living with HIV disease unless one also thinks about the possibility of death. So thoughts about death and dying have to be balanced by thoughts about life and living. In this way, the counsellor switches the focus between the two in order to help the patient to live better with HIV disease. An extract from an interview illustrates this:

Patient: The doctors have told me that my CD4 cell count is dropping and I feel very nervous about the future.
Counsellor: What are you most nervous about?
Patient: I suppose most about dying.
Counsellor: What aspects of living are you nervous about?
Patient: Having to face my parents with this news.

Counsellor: If they were here today, do you think they would agree that you need to be nervous?

Patient: That's a good question. I'm actually not sure.

Counsellor: What would they think you need to be nervous about, if anything, if they understood more about your illness?

Patient: That the way I may die may be unpleasant.

Counsellor: How do you think you might begin to discuss this with them?

Individual system and wider systems

Patients will often present themselves as the locus of the problem. They may describe the problems that they have in coping and adapting to living with HIV disease as being personal. The counsellor, by contrast, may have the view that these problems have implications for the wider system, comprising doctors, nurses and other professional and non-professional workers. Thus, when the patient talks about personal problems, such as depression, the counsellor may help him to think about the implications of this in his relationships with other people. Similarly, when he patient describes problems that he is having with other people, the counsellor will need to address their impact on the patient, as illustrated below:

Patient: I'm finding that my boyfriend is becoming more concerned about himself than he is about me.

Counsellor: What does he do that gives you this idea?

Patient: He's starting to spend more time with other people.

Counsellor: What effect does having less time to spend with him have on you?

Patient: I have more time to worry about my illness.

Counsellor: OK, are there any advantages to your having more time to yourself?

Patient: A few.

Counsellor: Such as?

Patient: It gives me time to think how I am going to reorganize my life, I read more and I get to see more of my parents.

Openness and secrets

Many patients fear the ostracism and social stigma that may result from their diagnosis. For this reason they may seek to keep it secret. In some circumstances, secrets may interfere with co-ordinated patient management and care. The tension between secrecy and the openness which may be needed for effective patient care is often discussed in sessions. The following conversation illustrates this point:

Patient: I guess everything I tell you in counselling is in strict confidence and you won't tell anyone.

Counsellor: What do you understand by confidentiality?

Patient: That no one other than you should know my diagnosis.

Counsellor: How do you think it might affect your treatment in hospital if ever you were to become ill?
Patient: It may make it more difficult for the doctor treating me.
Counsellor: Can you think of any particular problems that may arise?
Patient: I may be given the wrong drugs.
Counsellor: How might it benefit you then if more people knew?
Patient: Well, obviously there may be some advantages, but it depends *who* it is that knows.

Wanting to know and not wanting to know

Often patients will say that they want to know about the results of clinical tests, investigations or other procedures. In reality, however, they may not want to know or they may be ambivalent. This problem may never be entirely resolved. Patients, and indeed members of the health care team, may have different views about how much information about the patient should be made known. For this reason, there is often an ongoing discussion in the course of counselling about the management of information. This may lead to more open communication between the patient and the professionals caring for him.

Hope and hopelessless

With HIV disease, there is always a tension between feelings of hope and hopelessness. These feelings are directly linked to the complements of certainty and uncertainty. The counsellor may seek to maintain the patient's hope in the face of his life-threatening illness. This is not easily done. The counsellor can perhaps offer hope in relation to small goals, and at the same time not deny the reality that the possibility of illness is ever-present. As long as there is some uncertainty, there is an element of hope. The course or outcome of illness can never be accurately predicted. Certainty can also create some hope. A patient may be relieved that some of his symptoms can be diagnosed and promptly treated after receiving a positive HIV test result, which was not the case before he had his test. Clearly, the converse is also true and uncertainty may erode a patient's feelings of hope in other situations. The complements of hope and hopelessness are introduced in the example below:

Patient: I feel quite hopeless now that I've been given this positive HIV test result.
Counsellor: In what areas do you see some possible hope?
Patient: That major advances may be made in the medical field that could perhaps prevent further deterioration in my condition.
Counsellor: What could you hope for in more personal areas, for example, family and friends?
Patient: That my friends show me that they care for me.
Counsellor: What would you start noticing if this were to occur?

Temporal themes

At any one moment in counselling a particular time period is being referred to. A patient may, for example, say that he is currently depressed. The counsellor may then examine at least two other time periods. The first would be the past. The counsellor may ask the patient whether he has felt depressed in the past and how he coped with that. He may also ask him, in thinking about the future, what would happen if he continued to feel so depressed and these feelings never went away, or how things would look if his depression were to lift. In this way, the counsellor can always introduce a new view of the problem with a temporal theme. For example:

Patient: I have felt so depressed for the past two weeks.
Counsellor: When last did you feel so depressed?
Patient: About two years ago.
Counsellor: What were the signs to you then that you were feeling less depressed?
Patient: I started to work more productively and wanted to socialize more.
Counsellor: How will it be different or the same when this bout of depression starts to lift?
Patient: Pretty much the same.
Counsellor: And if it takes longer to lift, who will be aware that it's a longer period than usual for you?
Patient: John.
Counsellor: And did he have any concerns for you when you were depressed before?

Family dilemmas

The patient's ideas about what his family of affiliation (social) or family of origin (biological) might think about a particular problem should be discussed. He may already know their views or he may be asked to imagine them. This helps to place a problem in the context of relationships and gives the patient a new reference point from which to look at it. An excerpt from a counselling session follows:

Patient: My boyfriend feels that I am too ill to continue working.
Counsellor: What does he think you should do when you've stopped?
Patient: Just stay at home and rest.
Counsellor: Who agrees with him?
Patient: I think my parents both disagree.
Counsellor: Why do they think you should continue working?
Patient: They think it will take my mind off my troubles if I'm occupied or busy.
Counsellor: And what does your boyfriend think will occupy your thoughts while you are resting at home?
Patient: Perhaps how we can continue to care for each other in the difficult times ahead.

Dependence and abandonment

The nature of disease progression in HIV infection is such that there will be times when patients are satisfactorily able to look after themselves out of hospital, and other times when they will need to be in hospital. This may present as a dilemma in the context of counselling as some patients may resent being dependent on clinical care or even coming to counselling sessions. On the other hand, they may simultaneously express a fear of being on their own or indeed of being abandoned. This dilemma can be played out through contradictory messages given to the counsellor or other members of the health care team. It is not always necessary for the counsellor to interpret this back to the patient, but perhaps to be aware of the tension between abandonment and dependence. For example:

Patient: I really don't think it's necessary for me to be here today.
Counsellor: How is that different from the last time you were here?
Patient: Then I felt really sick and needed somebody to talk to and answer questions for me.
Counsellor: What sorts of things do you think you might want to talk about during well periods?
Patient: Perhaps if I could get more involved in my relationship while I was feeling better.
Counsellor: What do you think you would need to do in order to get more involved in your relationship?
Patient: Perhaps I should see you less when I am feeling better.

Separateness and involvement

These dilemmas are similar to those of dependence and abandonment. When a patient becomes ill and understands the possible implications of his illness, he may wish to live more separately from others. This may be, for example, because he may not want to risk infecting a sexual partner or because there may be a fear that a partner will desert him. On the other hand, at a time of crisis, the patient may feel a real need for a significant relationship and for close emotional involvement. A similar process may occur in the course of counselling where patients either do not want to keep appointments or may ask for more frequent appointments. For example:

Counsellor: When do you think you will have more worries or ideas to talk about with me: when you are sick or well?
Patient: It may vary.
Counsellor: If you were not to keep a future appointment would you expect me to think that you had nothing to talk about or that it was perhaps too difficult for you to talk about some issues just then?
Patient: I think that I couldn't face the upset of talking about certain issues.

Change and preservation

One of the counselling goals is to help people adapt and change, and at the same time preserve healthy behaviours. This goal addresses the therapeutic balance. The counsellor constantly processes language which may include some of his ideas about the following: What is the patient telling me? What is a problem? What does the patient system want changed? What does it want conserved? In keeping with the counselling task, the counsellor may try to generate considerable change, which in turn may throw the therapeutic system out of balance. Through responding to the feedback, the counsellor can redress the balance by identifying whether the patient is growing emotionally or whether he has become stuck. In the face of the latter, the counsellor should ask himself: 'Am I pushing for change when change is not wanted? Am I trying to change the system in a way that is inappropriate?' The following example addresses the problems of change:

Patient: I feel very confused about my life now that I'm so ill.
Counsellor: I realize that there are so many aspects of your life that you would like to change. Are there any aspects that you would like to keep the same?
Patient: How my parents look after me.
Counsellor: What does your boyfriend think you'd like to change most?
Patient: The fact that I have so little energy to participate properly in our relationship.
Counsellor: What would he most likely want to keep the same?
Patient: That I won't ever feel like leaving him.

CONCLUSION

Some of the more challenging problems in clinical practice stem from rigid beliefs and the management of bad news or feelings of hopelessness. A systemic approach recognizes that these problems can present between patients, family members, close contacts and members of the health care team. In this chapter, an approach has been described for initiating counselling in relation to patients' belief systems which may indicate that they have choices in how they view their relationships and what may be happening to them. This is not to suggest that by creating balance in difficult clinical situations, patients will be completely relieved of their problems. Balancing techniques are a first step towards reframing a belief or a problem. There may be some personal advantage, for example, in being in hospital as it may encourage the patient to be more open about his illness which he felt he could not be while he was still in good health. Complementarity can also be introduced into counselling by asking hypothetical and future-orientated questions such as: 'You complain that the doctors only seem to give you bad news. What might have to happen for them to be able to give you good news? How do you think that good or bad news would affect how you see your illness and your relationship with your doctors?'

There are potential problems for the counsellor in using the approach described in this chapter, and its use requires care and delicacy. A counsellor without training in this approach may use this technique as a means of avoiding the confrontation of problems with patients when this may be appropriate. Without supervision, the counsellor could inadvertently disqualify the patient's negative feelings and become combative with him by insisting on the 'good' side.

PART TWO

CLINICAL APPLICATION

SEVEN

The Role of Counselling in Pre- and Post-HIV Antibody Testing

'Where shall I begin, please your Majesty?' he asked. 'Begin at the beginning,' the King said, gravely, 'and go on till you come to the end: then stop.'

Lewis Carroll

INTRODUCTION

Pre- and post-HIV antibody test counselling is an essential part of the necessary range of psychological assessment and interventions in HIV care and treatment (Carballo and Miller, 1989). Counselling for an HIV test is given particular emphasis in this book because the issues it raises cover a wide range of the psychological, social, and medical implications of HIV infection. We have learned from our clinical and teaching experience that the skills needed to counsel people effectively before and after an HIV test enable health care providers to tackle some of the problems encountered at later stages of the illness. In addition, if the patient has had a satisfactory experience of pre- and post-test counselling, this may directly influence his view of counselling at all other stages of investigation and illness.

HIV testing in the 1990s will inevitably become more widespread and even a routine part of clinical diagnosis and treatment. The World Health Organization and a number of countries, including the United Kingdom, have recognized the far-reaching implications of HIV for the individual. Counselling is recommended both before blood is taken, and when the test result is given. The specific aim is to ensure that informed consent is given before testing (WHO, 1990), and that the patient receives psychological support afterwards. This chapter describes the background to HIV antibody test counselling and offers a procedure for counselling people about the test and giving results. Some guidelines for pre- and post-HIV antibody test counselling are suggested. Readers are referred to our book *AIDS: A Guide to Clinical Counselling* (Miller and Bor, 1988) for a more detailed and extensive description of how to counsel at pre- and post-HIV testing stages.

WHAT IS THE HIV ANTIBODY TEST?

The test for HIV antibodies is a diagnostic indicator of whether an individual has been infected with HIV. It alone does not indicate or predict whether, or when, that person will develop AIDS, although an increasing number of HIV-infected people are likely to develop AIDS over time. At present, cohort studies indicate that it takes on average 8 to 10 years before 50 per cent of HIV-infected individuals will develop clinical symptoms, although treatment, age and co-factors influence this (Moss and Bacchetti, 1989).

The test was first introduced in 1985. Initially, many people, including some health care professionals, considered that there was little reason to test for HIV, as not much could be done for people if they were found to be HIV-positive. Attitudes towards testing are likely to change as more effective primary and secondary treatments become available, and as the social stigma associated with HIV infection decreases. The decision to have an HIV test is complex and we do not have views about its use in individual cases. Ultimately, the decision to test depends on the doctor's clinical judgement and the patient's personal views and psychological circumstances.

Reasons for counselling

There are several reasons why counselling should accompany this test, even though many other tests are carried out without the patient's explicit consent. First, HIV infection, unlike some other conditions, can be passed on sexually; from mother to child perinatally, during delivery and postnatally through breast-feeding; and through blood and other body fluids (see Chapter 17). Counselling provides an opportunity to educate people about these risks of transmission and to promote behaviour change that will prevent the further transmission of HIV. The lives of those found to be HIV-positive can be profoundly affected.

Counselling can help people to make informed decisions by considering the advantages and disadvantages of being tested for HIV. They may also be better prepared emotionally for some of the possible personal and emotional consequences. Before a decision is made about testing it is important to know how the patient perceives the advantages and disadvantages of having the test. Even if he is asked, the counsellor's personal views about testing should not be discussed with patients, as they are inappropriate. However, too much discussion about the pros and cons of testing can confuse the patient and make decisions more difficult. The counsellor should supply information if the patient fails to touch on any issue that might be of particular importance for him. Listed below are some of the arguments for and against HIV testing.

1 MEDICAL TREATMENT AND CARE

The HIV antibody test is diagnostic for HIV infection. If people are aware of their HIV antibody status they can decide whether to seek clinical monitoring and care, where this is available. Having an HIV test is the first step in an assessment process, and a baseline from which the results of other predictive and diagnostic

ests can be used to determine the stage of HIV disease (see Chapter 8). The HIV
est alone does not give sufficient information on which to decide about treatment
or clinical care. Once the HIV infection has been diagnosed, decisions can be made
about treatments and care.

2   REDUCTION AND PREVENTION OF TRANSMISSION

HIV testing will enable those who are at risk of transmitting infection to be
informed and counselled on the prevention of transmission.

3   DECISION-MAKING IN RELATIONSHIPS

Some people request an HIV test before making decisions about entering into new
relationships, establishing more permanent relationships, or having children. A
positive result can reveal secrets about the past, such as drug use, homosexuality,
bisexuality or undisclosed relationships.

4   MANAGEMENT OF STRESS

The stress of living with uncertainty about the diagnosis can be reduced. Even
people with a late diagnosis of HIV infection may benefit from testing and
counselling. Since some people who are found to be HIV-positive may experience
increased stress as a result of the test, they may require more opportunity to talk
about their concerns beforehand.

5   IMPLICATIONS FOR TRAVEL AND LIFE INSURANCE

Some countries now require visitors and immigrants to have an HIV antibody test
before issuing entry visas. Insurance companies may also require people to have an
HIV antibody test before issuing policies where they consider that an applicant has
been at risk or when large sums of money are involved. The use of testing for HIV
in order to exclude people or limit their mobility is controversial.

6   PLANNING SERVICES

By identifying those who are infected with HIV, epidemiologists can advise on the
extent of HIV surveillance required. This is vital information for those who plan
services and allocate resources.

WHO SHOULD COUNSEL ABOUT THE HIV TEST?

As HIV infection becomes more widespread, all doctors and other health care
providers should discuss HIV and AIDS with their patients as a part of the routine
medical consultation and differential diagnostic process. In addition, provision
should be made for specialist counsellors to help with those who may have specific
fears before giving informed consent to testing.

WHERE SHOULD COUNSELLING TAKE PLACE?

Sexually transmitted diseases clinics, drug treatment centres and haemophilia units have experience in providing such a service. There should also be access to HIV testing and counselling in diverse settings such as family doctors' surgeries, family planning and antenatal clinics, as well as maternal and child health centres. As HIV spreads to the heterosexual population, assumptions cannot be made about 'high-risk' groups since it is the *activity*, rather than the *risk group*, that determines risk for HIV. We have not singled out different groups in HIV pre- and post-test counselling, as the problems of HIV are essentially the same for everyone regardless of the route of transmission. We recognize, however, that the members of each group – for example, chemically dependent intravenous drug users – may have specific problems relating to their lifestyle. Some voluntary and statutory organizations may want to identify HIV counsellors who are able to discuss HIV testing with people. To do this effectively, links with testing sites and medical services must first be established.

GUIDELINES FOR PRE- AND POST-TEST COUNSELLING

Pre- and post-HIV test counselling is likely to be more effective if the counsellor is clear about the aims of the session, and if the discussion is focused and time-limited. The main aims of HIV antibody test counselling are:
- to identify and clarify people's concerns and their risk for HIV;
- to check their understanding of how HIV is transmitted, how transmission can be prevented, and the meaning of the antibody test;
- to help people make more informed decisions by weighing up the benefits and disadvantages for them of having the test;
- to help people consider what might be their greatest concern if they were either HIV-negative or HIV-positive;
- to provide them with information about the personal, medical, social, psychological and legal implications of being diagnosed either HIV-positive or HIV-negative;
- to help prepare people for difficulties they may face in the future and to provide support for them, their family and their contacts.

Confidentiality

Since counselling for the HIV test usually takes place in a clinical setting, the counsellor should explain his position in the health care team and the aims of the session. The patient should be informed that confidential counselling routinely accompanies the HIV antibody test. For a more detailed description of dealing with confidentiality see Chapter 10.

A conversation may be opened as follows:

I am Mrs R, a counsellor, and I work as part of the HIV team. We always talk to people before they have blood taken for the HIV antibody test. This is because it is important that you understand what this test is for, and what the possible implication of the result may be for you before you agree to have the test. We have about 30 minutes for this conversation, which will be confidential. Any concerns about your health which are raised might make it important to involve others in our health care team.

Identify the perceived HIV risk

The counsellor should gather information from the patient simply by asking him questions which make no assumptions about the reasons for testing, the patient's concerns and the risk of HIV. It is equally important not to define the problem until the patient has first done so himself (see Chapter 3). For example:

> What was it that made you decide to come for the test at this stage?

This illustrates how the counsellor can begin to assess what events or beliefs have precipitated his need for a test. HIV infection inevitably affects relationships. A conversation about relationships can be started by asking:

> Who else knows that you have come for the test today?
>
> Whose idea was it that you should have a test?

Identify the patient's perception of his main risks of HIV, and check his understanding of HIV transmission and prevention. The pre-test counselling session is a unique opportunity to translate the health education messages from the media and elsewhere into a personal discussion. By asking questions and helping people to be specific, misconceptions can be identified, and correct information can then be given. Some of the following questions can be asked:

> Can you tell me the ways that you know that HIV is transmitted?
>
> How do you think that you might have been infected with HIV?

'Sex' may mean different things to different people so it is important to explore the range of potentially risky activities.

> What do you mean by having sex? Do you mean cuddling, kissing, anal or vaginal intercourse? I need to have an understanding of the activity that you think was risky in order to help us to assess the risk.

HIV is transmitted in the following ways:
(a) Through infected semen, vaginal fluid or blood entering the body via the anus, mouth, vagina or a break in the skin.
(b) By sharing infected needles, syringes, skin-piercing instruments or sex toys.
(c) By transfusions of infected blood or blood products given before donor screening and heat treatment were introduced.
(d) From mother to baby, *in utero*, at delivery or after birth by breast-feeding.

Transmission of HIV infection can be prevented by:
(a) Avoiding unprotected penetrative vaginal, anal or oral intercourse.
(b) Using condoms, spermicide, diaphragm or cap with care.
(c) Using only clean needles, syringes or other equipment.
(d) Not donating blood if you consider that either you or your sexual partner have been at risk for HIV.

Information about the HIV antibody test

The counsellor should endeavour to find out what the patient understands about the HIV antibody test. The HIV test is only a first step in diagnosis and cannot itself determine whether a person has AIDS or how he has been infected. The following example of dialogue shows how the counsellor can discuss this with the patient:

Counsellor: Can you tell me what you know about the test?
Patient: Does it tell me that I have AIDS?
Counsellor: No, it is not a test for AIDS. It only tells us that you have been infected some time in the past. It does not tell us how long you have been infected with HIV.
Patient: So will I get AIDS?
Counsellor: We cannot be certain about that. There are other tests we can do to help us know more about how well your immune system is functioning.

In the course of counselling, the following information about the test should be passed on to the patient:

> It is a blood test to see if HIV antibodies have appeared in the blood.
> It is a marker of infection with HIV.
> It is not a test for AIDS.
> It does not predict *if* and *when* AIDS will develop.
> There is a 'window period' of six weeks to three months between exposure to HIV and the development of HIV antibodies. It is important to establish the time of the first and the last perceived risk.
> The time between blood being taken and the result being available should be made explicit.
> The results will only be given in person, not over the telephone or by letter.

The patient's knowledge of the meaning of either a negative or positive antibody test result should also be clarified. For example:

> What do you understand about a positive test result?

If the result is negative, discussion about the last risk and the 'window period' is particularly important. For example:

> As you say that you might have had a risk three weeks ago, we would advise you to be tested again in three months, and again at the end of six months.

The implications of testing

The implications for the patient, his close contacts and family should be discussed. Some of the advantages and disadvantages of being tested, described earlier in this chapter, should be introduced at this point. The patient's concerns, if any, should first be identified. The following questions can be used by the counsellor:

What do you see as the possible advantages and disadvantages of having the test?

What might be your greatest concern if you decide to have the test?

Is there anyone else who might be affected by your decision to have a test?

How will you deal with your fear of telling your partner that you have come for the test?

Preparation for the result

Patients must be prepared for the implications of both a positive and a negative result. No pre-test counselling is either adequate or complete until the patient has been prepared in some way for a positive test result. For example:

If your test were positive what might that mean to you?

What changes might it bring?

Unless a patient has symptoms, it is not essential to make an immediate decision about an HIV test, and he may need to be allowed more time to think about it. For example:

Counsellor: You say that on the one hand you think you would feel less anxious if you had the test and knew the result, but on the other hand you cannot face knowing the result if it is positive. What would help you to make up your mind?

Patient: If I was sure it would be negative, but I know that is not possible now.

Counsellor: How long do you think you will be able to put up with the stress of not knowing?

Patient: I don't know, as I keep thinking that I have AIDS. I have a friend who went through all this recently.

Counsellor: Does he know that you have come today?

Patient: No. I haven't told anyone.

Counsellor: Have you thought of talking to him about how he came to his decision?

Patient: I might tell him I am thinking of being tested.

Counsellor: As you are so unsure, I suggest you think about it a little more and we can meet again when you are ready to talk again.

Informing others

Discussion between the patient and counsellor should address whom the patient would *want* to tell, whom he *will* tell, and who he thinks *should* be told, such as friends, family, doctors, dentists and employers. Discussion could be opened by one or more of the following questions from the counsellor:

Whom would you want to tell if your result is positive?

You say that you do not want to tell your wife. What do you fear most about telling her?

What would make it easier to tell her?

Some patients are reluctant to discuss HIV with their family doctor, fearing a breach of confidentiality in the surgery or the disclosure to other family members who might also be patients of that doctor. However, patients should be made aware that if family doctors are not fully informed about their condition then they may not be able to offer appropriate treatment and care when they are consulted for symptoms which may be HIV-related, such as coughs and rashes. The inclination to keep the diagnosis from the family doctor needs to be balanced against some difficulties that may ensue in obtaining good medical and nursing care in the community.

Social support

It is important to explore the extent of the patient's social support. This is particularly relevant during the potentially stressful time between having the test and awaiting its result. Only realistic offers of professional contact should be made to avoid misunderstandings, as is illustrated below:

Between now and when you come for the results, if you have any questions or want to talk to one of the team, we are here between 9 a.m. and 5 p.m.

Should you not be able to talk to one of us, is there anyone else you could talk to until you are able to reach us?

Psychological assessment

Some form of global psychological assessment should be made before making decisions about HIV testing. This should be based on impressions of how the person might cope, and who else is around to provide emotional support. The counsellor needs to feel that the patient is making an informed decision and is not under any pressure from others to have the test. Some level of anxiety, distress and even agitation may be appropriate in response to a test. The patient should be reassured that many people feel some tense moments and have doubts about an important decision as such as this. For example:

How will you spend the time until you come back here for the result?

Is there anyone you will be with or will be able to talk to during this time?

Ending the session

Towards the end of the session the counsellor should make an opportunity for the patient to ask questions.

> Are there any questions you would like to ask, or anything that you would like to say that you have not had a chance to say so far during our talk?

The use of the phrase '. . . so far' prevents repetition and the risk of starting the discussion all over again. This can blur any clarity that has hitherto been achieved.

Before ending the session, clear arrangements must be made for giving the result. The patient may be prepared by saying:

> The result will be available on . . . at . . . (Avoid Fridays or times when there are fewer health care providers around to support the patient if necessary (Richards, 1986).) I will only give it in person, not on the telephone or in a letter. I always give the result as soon as you come into the room, whether it is negative or positive.

Post-test counselling

The post-test counselling interview, although separate from the pre-test counselling interview, is inextricably linked to it. The patient should have been prepared in some measure for a positive result. However, no matter how much discussion has gone on before the test, when the result is positive most patients are shocked. Many people may even forget the information discussed at the pre-test interview. They are often unable to absorb information after they have received the news, and some parts of the pre-test counselling interview may have to be repeated.

The purpose of the post-test counselling session is to give the result and help the patient to consider the implications for himself and others, in the immediate future and afterwards. For those found to be HIV-positive, it is important to convey some measure of hope, but at the same time not to give false reassurance.

Whenever possible the same person who counselled the patient at the pre-test stage should give the result. This is best given as soon as possible in order to use the time available to discuss the patient's concerns and to give information. For example:

> The result of your test is positive.

After a few seconds, if the patient is silent the counsellor can ask:

> What is the main thing on your mind now?
>
> Do you remember what a positive test result means?

After giving a positive test result, one counselling approach is to ask questions of the patient after a few moments in order to re-engage him after the initial shock. This prevents him from simply 'switching off' whilst the counsellor compensates for the distress or what may seem the erosion of hope by making long explanations. Assumptions should not be made, however, about the patient's possible reactions.

Some people are relieved by a positive test result as they can now understand their symptoms and no longer have uncertainty about the diagnosis. The positive result may also mean that the patient can decide to do something about previous health concerns. He may find the motivation to improve his diet or make certain priorities in his life. Conversely, he may not be overjoyed by a negative result as it may give rise to new problems in his life. He may, for instance, have to contemplate a sexual relationship that he had previously avoided because of the uncertainty about being infected with HIV. It is, however, of paramount importance to allow sufficient time for the patient to discuss concerns whether the result is positive or negative.

The meaning of the result

The patient's understanding of the result should be checked again, whether it is negative or positive. Stress, anxiety and confusion about the facts might impede the retention of the information.

Identify concerns and maintain hope

If the result is positive, the first step is to identify the patient's main concerns. If patients are helped to rank their concerns this may reduce their anxiety to manageable proportions. Both patient and counsellor will then feel less overwhelmed by a multiplicity of pressing issues. A positive HIV test result is the first step in investigating the patient's health. The counsellor should present available information about the tests and investigations, as well as explaining the possibilities for care and monitoring. To allay the patient's immediate fear that a positive result means AIDS and death, the counsellor can suggest that there is no reason to believe that this will happen immediately. For example:

Counsellor: You say that your concerns are about having AIDS, dying, telling your partner, losing your looks and your family. Which of those is the greatest concern to you right now?
Patient: Well, I suppose dying. I'm not ready to go yet.
Counsellor: What are the things that you still want to do?
Patient: Travel and have more time with my partner.
Counsellor: You tell me that you are feeling very well. An HIV test is only the first step in planning your care and treatment. Knowing your diagnosis does not change your present state of health and make you unable to do the things you have been doing.

If the result is negative it is equally important to check the patient's reactions and address any particular concerns. There may also be a need to return for another test to confirm the negative result.

Dealing with results

Patients may need the reassurance and support provided by knowing that their reactions and feelings may be entirely normal and that they can talk to members of the health care team should they wish. For many young patients this might have been their first experience of life-threatening adversity. The counsellor can help them to put their feelings into perspective. For example:

Patient: I feel so stupid just sitting here crying.
Counsellor: It seems to me an entirely normal response.
Patient: It all seems so hopeless.
Counsellor: I know it seems a crazy thing to say right now, but is there anything that you feel is not so hopeless?
Patient: I suppose so. At least I feel well, and perhaps there is still lots of time.

Medical care

Information about medical follow-up and treatments should be given either at this stage or when it is felt that the patient is ready to discuss this aspect of care. Giving this information helps to engender and maintain some feelings of hope. It is useful first to explore the patient's knowledge and perceptions about treatment and care before giving this information, as he may otherwise not take in what is being said.

What do you know about tests that can be carried out to monitor your health and immune functioning?

Do you know about any treatments that can be given to people who are HIV-positive?

Social support

HIV-positive patients should be helped to consider carefully whom they *want* to tell about the condition, who they consider *ought* to be told, as well as *what* and *when* to tell those people. For example:

Is there anyone you want to tell about this immediately?

The counsellor can help the patient to rehearse what might be said in difficult social situations. For example:

If you decided to tell your wife tonight about your test result, how might you begin the conversation?

Counsellors might at this time be particularly drawn to support the newly diagnosed patient who has not yet drawn on his support network, or who does not have one. This can lead to feelings of stress and 'burnout' in health care providers. After the counsellor has given a positive test result it is especially important to secure the patient's links with his usual social support networks by asking:

Who is there around that you could talk to, or who might help you if you needed it?

The counsellor should give the patient information about local support organiz-ations so that he can talk to others who have known about their diagnosis for longer. However, it should not be assumed that everyone either wants or would benefit from this type of contact.

Health education

The counsellor should engage the patient in discussion about preventing HIV transmission to others, as well as protecting himself from acquiring new infections that might further compromise his health. The counsellor should stress the importance of eating well and taking sufficient rest.

Period immediately after post-test counselling

After giving a positive result to a patient, it is important to find out what he might do for the next few hours or days, and how he sees himself coping. Some patients may become very distressed and a few may have suicidal thoughts. The following questions can be used to assess the patient's reactions and to give him some realistic links with professional help should he wish to use it:

Where are you going when you leave here?

Is there anyone you want to phone?

If you get very upset you can phone me during the next week, between 9 a.m. and 5 p.m. After hours you should go to Accident and Emergency, where they are able to call one of us if necessary.

You say that you are very distressed. How are you going to handle this?

Follow-up counselling

A follow-up appointment should always be offered in order to address issues that might not have been covered, and to reassure the patient that there will be time for further discussion and continued contact.

Ending the session

The counsellor should summarize what has been discussed in the session and highlight important areas covered or that need to be attended to in future meetings. For those with a negative result, it might be necessary to arrange a future testing time or to discuss how to avoid high-risk situations when infection might be transmitted. The counsellor should strike a balance between communicating the fact that at present HIV cannot be cured and imparting more optimistic information about the successful treatment of many associated infections.

CONCLUSION

Irrespective of the reasons for testing, counselling is vital to address some of the psychosocial sequelae of having an HIV test and the potential bad news of a positive result. A counsellor's views about the test may be influenced by his knowledge about HIV, the diagnostic and predictive indicators of HIV illness, the choices available to patients in his clinic or medical setting, and the latest developments for treatment. Many patients are now well informed about the possible benefits of early testing and want to discuss the implications of a positive result. Counselling patients about the test is a way of opening up communication between counsellors and patients. Counsellors thus lay the foundation for comprehensive medical and psychosocial care.

HAROLD BRIDGES LIBRARY
S. MARTIN'S COLLEGE
LANCASTER

EIGHT

Counselling Patients with HIV Infection about Laboratory Tests with Predictive Values

... the theorist can only build his theories about what the practitioner was doing yesterday. Tomorrow the practitioner will be doing something different because of these theories.

Reusch and Bateson

INTRODUCTION

Since the Human Immunodeficiency Virus was first identified in 1983 (Barre-Sinoussi *et al.*, 1983) there has been considerable research into the natural history of disease progression and factors associated with this in infected patients. A number of laboratory markers of immune function have been recognized as predictive indicators of disease progression (Moss and Bachetti, 1989). Patients may need to understand the implications of these tests if they are to make informed decisions about whether or not to enter clinical trials, accept prophylactic and primary treatment, or consider the options in their work and close relationships. It is therefore extremely important for counsellors to communicate information about laboratory tests.

The aim of this chapter is to describe how discussion about tests and investigations can help the clinical care of patients and to offer some suggestions for counsellors. The counselling about predictive values should initially be provided by a doctor, who may call on the help of a specialist counsellor.

SOME LABORATORY TESTS AND INVESTIGATIONS THAT MAY HAVE PREDICTIVE VALUE IN HIV INFECTION

The HIV antibody test was the first reliable marker of HIV infection used in health care settings and blood transfusion services. Other laboratory test results that, individually or in combination, can be regarded as prognostic markers of disease progression include absolute CD4 lymphocyte counts and HIV p24 antigen serostatus (Phillips *et al.*, 1991), raised levels of B2 microglobulin (Sifris and Sher, 1988), neopterin (Kramer *et al.*, 1988), and CMV IgG antibodies (Webster *et al.*, 1989). These tests vary in their predictive power. Sequential values are of more significance than single values alone. They are all blood tests which can be carried out regularly provided there are suitable clinical and laboratory facilities. Other invasive and non-invasive investigations which may yield important information about a patient's current state of health and prognosis include X-rays, CT and MRI scans, lumbar punctures, bronchoscopies and endoscopies. Some have clinical value alone, while others may yield insights into the patient's condition when combined with other tests.

Reasons for counselling about tests and diagnostic investigations

Counselling for laboratory tests and diagnostic procedures focuses on giving information. There are several main aims in counselling patients about tests and investigations:

1 To facilitate communication and understanding between the doctor and patient by providing an important opportunity to address sensitive or difficult issues that affect the patient's life and the doctor's management of the patient.
2 To improve the patient's understanding about specific tests being carried out to help him make informed decisions about the options for treatment and care, as well as about relationships and work.
3 To help the patient and, where appropriate, his close contacts understand his present stage of HIV disease and to prepare him for possible changes.
4 To address any specific anxieties about HIV infection at any particular stage, with a view to reducing this anxiety to manageable proportions.
5 To provide an opportunity to discuss drug trials and new treatments.
6 To convey a measure of hope to those whose HIV antibody test proves positive, by talking about advances in treatment.

The results of these laboratory tests may reveal 'hidden' manifestations of immunodeficiency. It is possible that the doctor may have hints of deterioration or bad news before the patient experiences the clinical symptoms of ill health. In contrast, overt clinical symptoms of disease, such as Kaposi's sarcoma, raised temperatures and general malaise, may be noticed by the patient without tests having to be carried out by the doctor. A failure to discuss these laboratory tests with patients may create misunderstandings and lead to an impasse between the doctor and patient, particularly where there are secrets or where patients are not adequately prepared for the outcome of tests which might suggest bad news (see Chapter 5).

It is important to facilitate direct and unamibiguous conversations about tests between patients, doctors and other health care staff. In certain circumstances doctors may be reluctant to discuss tests with their patients. They may fear that the consequence of this communication would be the erosion of hope and the creation of uncertainty for the patient.

PSYCHOLOGICAL IMPLICATIONS OF TESTS AND INVESTIGATIONS

The patient's changing clinical condition has implications for his emotional and psychological well-being and for his interpersonal relationships. These changes and their implications are discussed below and are illustrated by conversations between the patient and counsellor.

Change and transition

The results of laboratory tests and diagnostic procedures may represent change and transition. The transition from one clinical stage of the disease to the next results in changes in the psychological as well as the physical state of the patient. For some this may be a source of increased stress. New adjustments may have to be made and psychological equilibrium re-established. A number of physical, social and emotional changes occurring over a short period may have a profound psychological impact on the patient. He may have adjustment problems, for instance, with treatment compliance, family relationships or social support. These problems may present to counsellors as psychological symptoms including depression, panic attacks or emotional blunting. The following extract from a conversation illustrates how the introduction of treatment allows the discussion of a changing view of illness.

Counsellor: How might taking AZT affect your view of living with HIV?
Patient: It is a big change for me. It makes me realize I actually could become ill. It will probably remind me that I have HIV each time I take a pill.
Counsellor: How do you think you will cope with this change?
Patient: In the way I usually do. Just get on with it, and, over time, I guess I'll get used to it.

Certainty and uncertainty

Tests with predictive values may create certainty where there was previously uncertainty. Assumptions should not be made about how individuals might respond to greater or lesser degrees of certainty. For some patients uncertainty can mean greater hope whereas for others the certainty that they have AIDS may enable them to face each day at a time more easily. Certainty and uncertainty in HIV can never be mutually exclusive. While there may be certainty that over time the majority of people with HIV infection will develop symptoms, the nature and course of the disease for the individual remains uncertain (Lefere *et al.*, 1988).

Equally, even if a patient has a full battery of predictive tests indicating that disease is imminent, one can never be certain when he will become ill, and with which infections.

CASE EXAMPLE F: Restoring a balanced view of the future

David, a 25-year-old homosexual man, came to have an HIV antibody test after many months of worrying that he might be infected with HIV. The result was positive and David's reaction in the post-counselling session was despondency about the future. The doctor did not want to let David leave without giving him some reason for hope. He feared that the man might become so despondent that he would kill himself. The doctor introduced the idea of hope by referring to the laboratory tests which would accompany his follow-up care and treatment. David had said that the main thing on his mind was that he was going to die. The doctor could have explored the patient's main fears and concerns about dying, but chose to try to instil some hope and restore the balance that had been disturbed by the news. This brief extract from the mid-point in the session demonstrates how the doctor introduced the subject to a newly diagnosed man who was in shock:

Counsellor: David, what do you know about available treatments to help you?
David: Nothing, I know there is no cure and I will die.
Counsellor: There is no cure, but there are things that can be done now to help your quality of life. Have you heard about any of the tests we do to help us decide what is the best treatment to give you and when to give it?
David: I've read something about T cells.
Counsellor: Yes, we can measure how your immune system is working so we can try to help you decide about treatments, or drug trials, if these are appropriate. We do this as a routine during your follow-up care. We can treat and prevent some infections such as pneumonia.
David: I didn't know that.
Counsellor: How much do you want to know about the tests that we do?
David: I'm not sure right now. I suppose I need to know a bit more, and I will get used to this after I've had time to think.
Counsellor: Next time we meet we can discuss this more. Meanwhile, if there is anything else you think about once you have left me, you can also speak to Sister Oliver who will be taking your blood.

Beliefs affecting different meanings attached to test results

Doctors, counsellors and patients may attribute different meanings to predictive values. Increased quality control of the tests may, for example, affect people's beliefs about their effectiveness. Patients may focus on their social and personal circumstances, whereas counsellors may focus on psychological health and doctors on the physical health and treatment possibilities. An example illustrates this:

Patient: I find it hard to believe that the tests you do are completely accurate.
Counsellor: What do you know about how we monitor the quality and reliability of the tests?
Patient: Not much, but I suppose what matters to me is if I feel well. I do not like thinking about the future.
Counsellor: Do you want me to continue to tell you the results of tests?

Patient: You can go on doing them, but I'm sceptical about the results.

Counsellor: It would be hard for me to continue providing the best care that I can without the guidance of the results of the tests, but how you feel in yourself is also important.

Secrecy

Decisions about when, what and how to give patients potentially upsetting information is central to the HIV patient's effective clinical and psychological management. A falling CD4 count may, for example, be withheld to *protect* the patient from additional anxiety and stress, but at the same time may place more responsibility on the doctor. Discussion with the patient about what he wants, or may not want, to know from tests can help to avoid the misunderstandings that can arise from withholding information. It can also avoid forcing potentially disturbing information on to those patients who might either be psychologically unready or unable to cope with such information. For example:

Doctor: Let us decide how we should proceed for the next few months. What do you want me to do about the test results?

Patient: You can do them, but only tell me when you think I have to know.

Doctor: What things do you think you really ought to know?

Patient: If you think the time has come when I have AIDS.

Doctor: If I had results that made me think I should offer some treatment, perhaps to prevent you getting an infection, what should I do?

Patient: Then you would have to tell me.

When to talk to patients about laboratory tests and investigations

Discussion can take place at any stage of contact with the patient, based on an assessment of the patient's mental state and behaviour. Three possible counselling options for dealing with difficult situations have been described in detail in Chapter 5. The tests can be done *without* discussion with the patient. This avoids raising issues of uncertainty and change. The doctor may then take the chance of keeping the concern about falling CD4 lymphocyte counts to himself. Secondly, the discussion of difficult issues, such as falling CD4 counts, which indicate a vulnerability to illness, can be *postponed*. The risk of doing this is that the patient might become ill, for example with *Pneumocystis carinii* pneumonia, without prophylactic treatment having been offered. This could be considered negligent in the light of current medical knowledge. A third option is to talk about these tests at an *early stage* when the patient is well and follow-up care is being planned. Hope can be more easily maintained early on by giving information about available treatments.

CONCLUSION

Discussion about laboratory tests should ideally be included in the on-going conversations between the patient and the doctor. Many decisions about treatment and care can be shared between the patient and health care professional. An atmosphere can then be created in which important information about the patient's condition can be discussed with him when appropriate. Counselling about the interpretation of laboratory values and the associated fears that might arise from the test results might help people to face both the uncertainty and certainty of their illness more adaptively and enable them to live more positively with HIV . The provision of counselling about predictive values depends on the setting and the availability of tests and counselling expertise. Investing time in counselling about tests from the outset may reduce the need for crisis counselling at a later stage. The need to address the broader psychological issues of change and transition, hope and hopelessness, certainty and uncertainty exists in every clinical and counselling setting in which HIV patients are cared for.

NINE

The Role of Focused Counselling for Drug Trials

'What is it you want to buy?' the Sheep said at last, looking up
for a moment from her knitting.
'I don't quite know yet,' Alice said, very gently. 'I should like to
look all around me first, if I might.'
'You may look in front of you, and on both sides, if you like,'
said the Sheep: 'but you can't look all round you – unless
you've got eyes at the back of your head.'

Lewis Carroll

INTRODUCTION

More effective treatments and vaccines for HIV are becoming increasingly likely. Drug trials are an essential feature of medical practice which continually seeks to offer better treatments to patients. We have to rely on clinical drug trials and post-mortem examinations to assess the efficacy of treatments. This chapter highlights some aspects of counselling about clinical drug trials for people with HIV disease. It describes a counselling approach which can be incorporated into the medical consultation process at different stages of a trial.

In order to obtain the patient's informed consent it is obligatory to explain to patients the aims and purpose of a clinical trial, the conditions for entry and remaining in the trial, and any possible side effects of the treatment. The social and emotional effects of being in a trial are less often given consideration, yet these may have significant implications for compliance with, and adherence to, the trial protocol and for the general well-being of the patient. Drug trial-related counselling will inform patients about the aims of the trial and improve the collaborative relationships between the doctor and patient, whether or not the patient opts to enter into the trial. Our experience gained from counselling patients in the Concorde MRC/Inserm (United Kingdom and European) trial of Zidovudine for asymptomatic patients with HIV infection is used to highlight some of the main counselling issues.

THE CONTEXT OF DRUG TRIALS IN HIV DISEASE

In the absence of tried and proven treatment, many patients are willing to try a course of treatment of an experimental drug in the hope of deriving some benefit not otherwise available. Furthermore, many patients with HIV disease are well informed about treatments and new developments. Doctors are willing to offer trial opportunities whenever appropriate, thus providing some measure of hope to their patients.

The way in which drug treatments are perceived by patients inevitably affects their recruitment and compliance. Both patients and clinicians will have views about drug trials, approached from different angles. *Patients* may hold views about trials, medication in general, or about a particular drug, as was the case with Zidovudine. In 1988, recruitment for the Concorde I trial was complicated by patients' perceptions about the toxicity and efficacy of Zidovudine. These perceptions were gleaned from the results of previous trials where the drug was used in large doses for symptomatic patients with a diagnosis of AIDS. Some patients were concerned about the possible side effects of the drug. The offer of Zidovudine through the trial could be seen as a last therapeutic effort in a clinical situation that was potentially hopeless. Perceptions like these have to be taken into account.

The meaning of trials for the *clinician* may also influence his approach to recruitment and follow-up. Enlisting patients to clinical trials can be seen as an important contribution towards research and may enhance the reputation of the participating team. Thus, in some instances, there might be pressure on doctors to recruit patients resulting in pressure on them to join trials. In some settings, the participation in drug trials may be the only chance of obtaining a drug or the clinical monitoring that might otherwise not be available. Drug trials might be a way of increasing staff with research doctors and nurses. Lastly, from the point of view of the patient–doctor relationship, a doctor might feel that he is helping the patient by entering him in a trial.

In some countries and settings drug trials may not be available. Voluntary organizations such as 'ACT UP', among others, which keep a watchful eye on the moral and ethical rights of patients, have been instrumental in ensuring that the results of trials are rapidly disclosed and published. These organizations have challenged the pace of drug trials, the possibility of patient access to trials, the agendas for drug-related research and the early release of new drugs.

PSYCHOLOGICAL AND PRACTICAL IMPLICATIONS OF CLINICAL TRIALS

The more common issues pertaining to clinical drug trials are practical considerations, time and motivation, beliefs in traditional medicine and trials, relationships with health care providers, and psychological stability.

If the psychological and practical implications of participating in drug trials are taken into account, patients are more likely to be willing to join trials and adhere to the protocols. In addition, information about the trial, its conditions and restraints, must be clear and unambiguous. If potential problems are identified at an early stage, the patient is then more prepared for some of the possible outcomes of entering the trial, should he choose to participate. These are discussed below.

Practical considerations

Practical constraints on time, payment of fares and permitted absence from work may prevent some patients from entering into a trial and may affect the participation of others who do enrol. The trial research team is responsible for ensuring that undue stress and demands are not placed on patients who opt to participate in the trial by reducing waiting times and efficiently organizing the clinical and laboratory follow-up. Practical considerations such as these enhance the chances of patients remaining in the trial; they also help to ensure more meaningful outcomes since data are then collected regularly and reliably.

Time and motivation

Entering a drug trial involves a commitment of time and motivation on the part of patients. Misunderstandings over practical and psychological difficulties can be reduced if the patient's reasons for joining the trial are understood and respected.

Beliefs

The beliefs patients have about being in a trial should be considered, as they are closely linked to their motivation for entering and remaining in the trial. Some patients may equate trials with experimentation and research, and resent being human 'guinea pigs'. Others view trials as an opportunity to do something about their medical condition which they might otherwise feel was beyond their control. Yet others are willing to enter trials for altruistic reasons, considering that they may help future generations of HIV-infected patients. Inaccurate interpretations of key words lead to misunderstandings. For example, some patients may not understand the concept of a placebo and believe that all pills are a definite treatment.

Perceptions of having HIV infection

Entering a drug trial is likely both to be influenced by, and to influence, a patient's perceptions of having HIV. For those who cope with HIV by avoiding thinking about it, entering a trial and the associated regular medical surveillance and tablet-taking are a constant reminder of the disease.

Relationship with health care providers

The patient's participation in drug trials may affect his relationship with health care providers in different ways. Some patients may feel unable to refuse participation, and may subsequently find ways of 'opting out' by not attending for appointments or reporting unfavourable side effects. There may seem to be a different level of care and attention for those in and out of the trial. Patients may need to be reassured that, if they are not participating in the trial, their care will not in any way be compromised. They will need particular reassurance if they have a good, but dependent, relationship with their doctor but fear the repercussions of not pleasing him by entering the trial.

Psychological stability

The opportunity to enter a drug trial can present a series of challenges to the psychological stability of patients with HIV disease. The patient will have to make decisions about whether to enter the trial, whom he wants to tell about it and the explanation he will give to others. This is a transition which may upset the patient's capacity to cope. For some patients it may entail 'coming out' to family, friends and employers about a diagnosis or explaining the need for regular hospital attendance. Some may begin to see themselves as sick or unwell, which in turn may influence how others relate to them. Not only is the patient's self-image affected by a drug trial, but he may be under increased stress from uncertainties about possible side effects, about whether he is actually receiving the drug, or if the trial is of any value.

COUNSELLING TASKS IN RELATION TO DRUG TRIALS

Counselling for drug trials can be included in the medical consultation process at all stages of the trial. The following points summarize the information that needs to be communicated to help the patient decide whether or not he wishes to enter the trial:

- the reason why a certain drug is being investigated;
- what the therapeutic effect of the drug may be;
- any possible side effects of the drug;
- the criteria for entry;
- the length of the trial;
- required frequency of attendance at clinics for surveillance and monitoring;
- the specific monitoring tests and clinical examination required;
- the conditions for withdrawal from the trial;
- protocols for treatment and care if the patient becomes unwell during the trial;
- discussion of available options.

GUIDELINES FOR DRUG TRIAL COUNSELLING

A plan of relevant issues to explore at different stages of a clinical drug trial helps to keep counselling sessions focused. The number of follow-up counselling sessions necessarily depends on the length of the clinical trial. Suggested counselling sessions are at pre-enrolment, enrolment and thereafter at intervals of six or twelve months. Some examples of areas of discussion and questions will be given for each stage.

Pre-enrolment

1 PROVIDE INFORMATION

Information about the trial can be provided through individual discussion, written material, specific group meetings, or a combination of these (Lee, Miller and Goldman, 1989). Some examples of questions to open discussion include:

> I want to discuss with you the possibility of participating in a drug trial. I would like to offer you some information about the trial and an opportunity to ask questions before we ask you to consider whether or not you would be interested in the trial.

> What do you know about the available treatments for HIV infection and other associated infections?

> What do you understand about your current state of health?

Clarify the patient's knowledge about clinical trials in general and the particular trial in question. Explain the purpose of a placebo, if this is relevant. Avoid using technical words or jargon, such as 'double-blind placebo-controlled trial' or 'independent variable' to ensure complete understanding. Misunderstandings are less likely to occur if the patient's knowledge and views are first explored before giving new information. Long explanations more easily lead to misunderstandings, as the doctor has no way of checking the patient's knowledge. The following questions can be asked:

> What do you understand about a drug trial?

> What do you understand by the word 'placebo' as applied to a drug trial?

> What do you know about Zidovudine?

> Do you know why we are offering this trial to people who have HIV infection, but no symptoms?

2 ADVANTAGES AND DISADVANTAGES OF THE TRIAL

Provide an oppportunity to discuss the advantages and disadvantages of the trial by asking some of the following questions:

> What might be some of the advantages for you of being in the trial?

What do you think might be some of the difficulties you might face? How might you overcome them?

Who else will you discuss this with? What questions might they have?

The following is a summary of the main advantages and disadvantages of participating:

Advantages include:

The possibility of a drug being beneficial.

More frequent detailed medical surveillance to identify symptoms and provide treatment.

Being able to do something about HIV for oneself and future patients with HIV.

The opportunity for more general support and counselling.

Disadvantages include:

The possibility of side effects from the drug.

The fear that the drug could exacerbate symptoms or lead to a deterioration in health.

The inconvenience of frequent clinic or hospital visits.

A frequent reminder of HIV by having to take pills or attend for monitoring.

The uncertainty as to whether drug, placebo, a large or small dose is being taken, or whether resistance to the drug will develop.

The stress on relationships such as choosing whom to tell and not to tell, and the effort of perhaps secretly taking tablets.

Worries associated with having to withdraw for health reasons.

3 RELATIONSHIPS

The patient's close contacts can influence his decisions about enrolling, and his compliance with the trial protocol. These issues should be addressed with patients before entry into a drug trial and at all stages during the course of the trial. These questions help to address the issues:

What do you think your boyfriend's or parents' view of the trial would be?

If their view differed from your own, how would you handle this difference?

Would their views influence your decision about the trial?

4 ADDRESS CONCERNS

Addressing the patient's concerns can help to reduce misunderstandings about the trial, the effects of drugs, and the use of the results at the end of the trial. Some examples of questions that facilitate discussion are:

What might be your greatest concern about entering the trial?

If your partner or mother were here what would they say would be their greatest concerns?

You say that your main worry is that your colleagues at work will see you taking your pills. Is there any way that you think you could deal with that?

You tell me that the hardest aspect for you is feeling forced to think about HIV each time you take the tablets. What is it that helps you to continue to take them?

5 ADDRESS THE BELIEFS

The patient's beliefs and motivation for entering into the trial should be considered. Some questions that the counsellor can ask to open up discussion of this aspect include:

How might participating in the trial affect your view of having HIV?

How might your choice not to participate affect your view of having HIV?

6 WITHDRAWING OR BEING WITHDRAWN FROM THE TRIAL

Early discussion of having to withdraw from the trial for any reason can help the patient to be more prepared for this possibility. It can also help to reduce staff stress when, for instance, they have to communicate the bad news of withdrawing patients from the trial because of side effects or a change in the patient's clinical condition. If the patient's beliefs about being withdrawn from the trial are understood, they can be addressed in counselling. Patients may think 'This is the end of the road' or 'I'm OK: the drug isn't.' Some examples of questions to identify the beliefs are:

How might you react if you had to stop the trial because it seemed that the medication was adversely affecting you?

If for any reason you wanted to stop participating in the trial, who would you tell, and would you foresee any difficulties in discussing it with us?

7 ENDING THE SESSION

Ending the interview with a summary of the main points discussed, and an assessment of the patient's suitability for the trial, clarifies the position for the patient and doctor. No patient should be under pressure to sign up for a trial 'on-the-spot'. The patient should be allowed time to consider the implications of the trial after a first interview and encouraged to bring questions to the next meeting.

Enrolment

1 REVIEW HOW DECISIONS WERE MADE

Identifying the factors that influenced the patient's decision about the trial helps to increase understanding of his motivation. It is important to maintain a neutral stance and not to indicate that the patient has in any way compromised his future care by enrolling or refusing to enrol. Some examples are listed below:

What helped you to make the decision to participate in the trial?

As you have decided not to participate in the trial, what influenced you most in making this decision? If you changed your mind for any reason would you feel able to approach us?

2 KNOWLEDGE ABOUT THE TRIAL

The counsellor should give the patient another opportunity to confirm his understanding about the trial. For example:

> Before starting the trial, can you clarify for me once again your understanding of the aims of this trial?

3 PRE-EMPT DIFFICULTIES AND ENHANCE COMMUNICATION

To pre-empt difficulties is one way of enhancing communication between doctors and patients. For example:

> If you felt, for any reason, during the trial that you were unable to adhere to the requirements, who would you tell, and what would you do about it?

> Do you think that anyone would be surprised or disappointed if you decided to withdraw from the trial?

Six-monthly review

1 REVIEW CONCERNS AND PRACTICAL PROBLEMS

After six months on a trial difficulties should be identified by the counsellor. For example:

> Has being on the trial affected your day-to-day life in any way?
> What changes, if any, have you or others noticed?
>
> Who else knows that you are in this trial?
>
> Now that you have been participating in the trial for six months, what might be your main concern?

Patients should be given an opportunity to express their views about the trial. For example:

> If you were to choose again about the trial, would you make the same choice?
> Would your partner or family have any other views?

Ask the patient about practical aspects of the trial in order to assess his compliance. The questions should be asked in a neutral, non-judgemental way.

> Over the past few months how often have you forgotten to take your pill:
> – less than five times?
> – 5–10 times?
> – 20 times or more?
>
> How many follow-up appointments have you missed?
> What were the reasons for this?

2 PERCEPTIONS OF DRUG DOSAGE OR PLACEBO

Most patients, at different stages of the trial, will think about whether or not they are on the placebo. They may notice small changes by closely examining themselves. This should be considered normal, and patients should be reassured about what may seem to them obsessive behaviour. For example:

> How are you coping with not knowing whether you are on placebo or a high-dose drug?

> It seems perfectly understandable that you feel the need to keep checking yourself.

As time passes, it is likely that the patient's compliance with the protocol and clinical follow-up will be influenced by his views about whether he is on a drug or placebo. Such difficulties may depend on the patient's motives for being in the trial. For example, if the patient enters the trial in the hope that he will receive treatment, compliance may become difficult if he believes that he is receiving a placebo. Nevertheless addressing the uncertainty of the trial drug is important. For example:

> We have no way of knowing whether you are on drug or placebo but you may have your own ideas about that.

End of trial

The end-of-trial assessment will depend on the conditions of the trial and the patient's state of health. The counselling will have to be linked to the patient's special conditions, such as being withdrawn because of illness, the side effects of drugs, or voluntarily. If the trial period has ended, the following steps become part of the counselling.

1 INFORMATION ABOUT RESULTS OF TRIAL

Patients should be consulted about whether or not they want to know the outcome of the trial. Assumptions should not be made that they will want to know all the details of the research. For example:

> Do you want us to let you know about the outcome of the trial?

> Do you want to know whether you were on placebo, or high or low dose?

Sometimes information about a trial is disseminated prematurely through the media. In these circumstances counsellors will have to address the questions and anxieties of patients before trials are completed.

2 THE PATIENT'S VIEWS OF PARTICIPATING IN THE TRIAL

The effect on the patient of being in the trial and his perception of having HIV should be considered.

> Has being in the trial in any way influenced how you have coped with HIV?

Some questions that help to elicit the patient's views are:

> What have been the most difficult aspects for you, your partner and other family members about being in the trial?

Has being in the trial had any benefits for you? Would your partner have the same view?

3   ENDING SUMMARY

Making a summary after hearing the patient's views helps to finish the contact over the trial and to show appreciation of the patient's participation. This summary should be based on the patient's views rather than on the assumptions of the health care provider.

CONCLUSION

Drug trials inevitably have an impact on both patients and staff. They are time-consuming for both. There is a change in the relationship between the patient and the health care workers when there is regular follow-up as part of a trial rather than as part of the monitoring of general health. Patients may feel that they are doing something for the health care provider. This aspect of their relationship cannot be ignored. More open communication facilitated by structured, focused interviews and questions makes patients more likely to remain on the trial. They can more readily accept being withdrawn from the trial if the possibility is indicated to them early. Health carers are likely to be less stressed if the discussions about the trial and possible problems are addressed before they occur.

Ultimately, counselling about drug trials is to help patients make informed decisions for themselves about whether or not to participate. The choice of whether to enter into a trial is the patient's, but it requires collaboration between the clinician and patient if patient management is to be enhanced.

TEN

Secrecy-related Problems in HIV Management

At last the secret is out, as it always must come in the end.

W.H. Auden

INTRODUCTION

Patients with HIV may present with problems that are psychological, yet they derive from the medical aspects of HIV. Foremost among these are problems of secrecy. This chapter sets out to highlight the significance of secrets in the clinical context and describes a counselling framework in which the management of secrets can be viewed. Some clinical situations are identified in which secrecy-related problems present and guidelines are offered for approaching the problem of secrets.

SECRETS AND CONFIDENTIAL INFORMATION

There is a difference between secrets and confidential information. Secrecy means the keeping of information from others (unless it is a shared secret), while confidential information, in the context of HIV, is a shared secret, perhaps within a sub-system of the health care team. The extent to which the secret has been shared is not always easy to distinguish. When a secret is finally revealed, an interested person may declare that he had well-founded suspicions about its existence. Problems may arise where those who feel it is their right to be informed suspect that certain information has been suppressed.

Frameworks for problem-solving and decision-making in some of these difficult cases have been described elsewhere (Bayer, Levine and Wolf, 1986; British Medical Association, 1987; Dickens, 1988; Gillon, 1987). Many of these problems concern patient consent for HIV antibody testing and ethical issues associated with the prevention of HIV transmission. Decision-making in relation to an HIV-infected psychiatric patient (Binder, 1987) is different from the decision a general practitioner must face when information about a patient's lifestyle is requested by an insurance company (Samuel, 1989). Secrets may even be the solution to some problems, for instance when a man chooses to hide his homosexuality from other family members to avoid being shunned by them. The implications of secrets will be discussed in the context of the clinical management of patients in the health care setting. It is not the intention in this chapter to offer a set of rules about where to safeguard secrecy, but to bring to light a frequent undercurrent that can impede the management of HIV patients, their partners and family.

CONCEPTUAL ISSUES

One of the most comprehensive accounts of secrets and their effects is by Karpel (1980), who examined this subject in the domain of family life. Many of these conceptual ideas are taken from his work. Secrets 'involve information that is either withheld or differentially shared between or among people' (p. 299). At least three major kinds of secrets can be described. *Individual secrets* are those in which one person keeps something private from others, be they members of the family, the health care team, or any other constellation of relationships. *Internal secrets* are different from individual secrets, in that one other person in the constellation of relationships keeps a secret from at least one other person. Lastly, *shared secrets* are shared between those inside a constellation of relationships, and information is kept from at least one other person or group outside. Examples of these are described below.

Examples of secrets

Individual secret   A married man keeps his worry about HIV to himself. He has recently lost weight, developed dermatological problems, feels tired and is increasingly breathless. He is worried about going to his general practitioner in case he suggests that he be tested for HIV.

Internal secret   At the start of their professional contact, an HIV counsellor says to his patient: 'Everything you tell me is confidential. I won't discuss it with anyone. Feel free to say whatever you want.'

Shared secret   After their son's death from HIV disease, a couple was faced with the problem of what to say to relatives. No one in the extended family knew the diagnosis. The son's diagnosis was shared only by his parents.

The 'power' (or burden) attributed to the secret-holder is but one social effect of a secret. Those who are excluded from knowing can be defined as being 'one down'. Loyalty, the fear of betrayal, self-protection, altruism and guilt over disclosure are all motives for secrecy which can set up particular dynamics in the interpersonal domain. The view that 'secrets = power' is simplistic. In fact, secrets can have the opposite effect on the patient when he experiences so much stress from their burden that he has anxiety-related symptoms such as diarrhoea, sweats, weight loss or exhaustion, which may be similar to symptoms of AIDS. Invariably, boundaries and alliances between people are either created, strengthened or destroyed by secrets. Their effects, therefore, are at all times structural, interactive, emotional and practical. The consequences of secrets are described below.

Consequences of secrets

Informational Deception, distortion, mystification, clarification.
Emotional Generation of anxiety, discomfort.
Relational Estrangements, violation of trust, protection, enabling people to get closer, creating new possibilities in relationships.
Practical Danger of unanticipated or destructive disclosure, accidental discovery, conserve or protect relationships.

(adapted from Karpel, 1980, pp. 299–301)

The effect of keeping any secret is seldom completely positive or negative. It is usually a combination of these, although to varying degrees. A secret may bring into focus themes associated with exclusion and dishonesty. At the same time, almost all secrets serve to protect someone from something. It is not uncommon, for example, for a young, newly diagnosed HIV patient to say to his doctor that he does not feel it would be wise to tell his ageing parents his diagnosis as they are in poor health. This may protect the parents at the cost of producing extreme anxiety for the patient. At the other extreme, an HIV-infected bisexual man who refuses to protect his wife, who is apparently unaware of his HIV status, creates a potentially hazardous situation and raises ethical dilemmas for those who share the secret. Keeping secrets may also be a symptom of other problems. People who choose not to disclose their HIV positivity at the time of donating blood may, among other problems, be denying their illness. Counselling can help patients to find more constructive ways of dealing with dilemmas and facing up to the consequences of more open communication with others.

Confidentiality and secrecy

Confidentiality and secrecy are related, but at times they are confused with one another. This can lead to misunderstandings in a clinical setting. Some members of health care teams resent not being told of a patient's HIV result, believing that the information is confidential to the whole team. Their colleagues might state that the matter is private and between themselves and the patient. In so doing they create a system in which there are secrets. They may justify this by laws pertaining to confidentiality in clinical settings. The context in which the secret is held cannot be separated from the nature of the confidential information nor from those participating in the social system created by the secret. For this reason, there will almost always be a variety of judgements about what constitutes confidentiality. While the Hippocratic Oath clearly states the doctor's duty not to disclose information that arises in the course of treatment, this privilege is not without exception or limitation, particularly where harm to the community outweighs confidentiality (Girardi, Keese and Traver, 1988). Discussion about these dilemmas, both within the clinical team and with the patient, is one step towards their management and solution.

Management of secrets

Health care professionals are not excluded from the effects of secrets, which can create considerable stress and lead to a feeling of being immobilized by the patient. Some may consider it their task to take sides, to advise patients or colleagues, or to expose the secret. Others may themselves generate secrets. After a patient has been given a positive HIV antibody test result, some doctors *prescribe* secrecy by suggesting to the patient that he does not tell anyone the result for fear of the stigmatizing reactions of others. Secrecy-related problems are inevitable, and health care workers may have both a personal and a professional view of how they should be managed. At times, these positions may be at variance with one another. A number of steps can be taken in order to minimize the sometimes harmful effects of this dislocation. These steps are at both the conceptual and executive levels and are derived from systemic theory (Andolfi, 1980; Hoffman, 1981).

Problem-solving for secrecy-related concerns

1 Identify whether there is a secret.

2 Identify whether there is a problem in relation to the secret, and for whom. Sometimes discussion about secrecy in general is sufficient to lead to the resolution of a secrecy-related problem.

3 Clarify the dilemmas involved in maintaining the secret. Balance should be attained between the advantages and disadvantages of maintaining the secret without the counsellor favouring a position. A range of possible outcomes should be discussed with the patient, using hypothetical and future-oriented questions (see Chapter 5).

4 There are several options available to the counsellor when faced with problems relating to secrets:
   (a) *Collusion:* agreement to preserve the secret.
   (b) *Challenge:* disagreement over keeping the secret; discuss the problems that arise for the counsellor in keeping a secret with the patient; the patient should be advised at the start of the counselling contact that it may not be possible for the counsellor to keep secrets that have legal implications.
   (c) *Opt out/refer:* where the secret does not have legal implications but creates an impasse in the therapy, the counsellor may suggest to the patient that he would prefer to refer him elsewhere.

A clinical case example is described next in which a potential impasse resulting from secrets is avoided.

CASE EXAMPLE G: Secrets in a difficult clinical situation

Thomas, a 29-year-old, HIV-positive, married bisexual man insisted that he would not tell his wife that he had come for an HIV test. The hospital doctor was concerned that Thomas's wife, if not already infected, was at risk of being infected by him. Before discussing the problem with the patient's general practitioner, the doctor decided to counsel Thomas about the implications of refusing to disclose his diagnosis. Future-oriented and hypothetical questions are often the key to breaking this all-too-common impasse in patient management and care.

Doctor: Thomas, if you were a doctor in my position, what would you think your patient should do?

Patient: I really don't care. There's no way I'm going to tell her. That would be the end.

Doctor: What might be the worst thing that would happen if you did tell her?

Patient: She'd probably leave me. I mean, she doesn't know I've had boyfriends. Anyway, I've got the kids to think about.

Doctor: Presumably you don't use condoms with your wife. What if she gets infected? Do you think she'd rather know now, while there's some chance she can prevent herself from becoming infected, or at a later point, when you or she, or maybe both of you, were ill? Who would you choose to look after your children?

Patient: I think she'd leave me and tell everyone about me. Also, she'd never let me see the kids.

Doctor: So which of those is the worst for you?

Patient: Perhaps if she left me. I don't know what I'd do. She's the one I'm going to need to keep me going.

Doctor: How might you cope if she did decide to leave you?

Patient: I've got a boyfriend I think I could stay with. Maybe he won't be interested in me any longer. Look, now I'm beginning to worry about my youngest kid too. Is it possible that he's also got it? Can you test him?

Doctor: Yes, we can test him. But what will you say to your wife about that?

Patient: I can see now it's better to tell her sooner rather than later. But I don't think I can face it alone. Will you tell her?

Doctor: Yes, if that's what you prefer. But first, let's think about how you might tell your wife. Then we can arrange to meet together with your wife and one of our counsellors. We can help all of you in the family to deal with this.

Conclusion

Secrecy-related problems are a recurring feature of the management of HIV-infected patients. In health care settings, they may arise between doctors and patients, patients and their families, and between health care workers themselves. Often, the limits of confidentiality are tested. It may be helpful to inform patients from the outset of the general limits of confidentiality. The American Psychiatric Association (1988) has provided helpful guidelines which apply to most clinical situations. These state that where another person's life is endangered by a secret, the counsellor may choose to disclose information that would protect a third party. For this reason, we do not say to patients that everything they say in the context of counselling will be kept secret between the counsellor and patient. We reserve the right to discuss important information with our colleagues, and the responsibility remains with the patient for what he chooses to disclose in a session. This may prevent the problem arising of whether or not to divulge secrets in the clinical setting.

A discussion between the patient and counsellor of the dilemmas incurred by secrets and their current and anticipated effects can remove a source of considerable stress from the relationship. It also returns to patients some of the responsibility for resolving problems. The use of future-oriented and hypothetical questions can help some patients to consider ideas and views that they might otherwise fear to address, in a non-confronting way. This can also reduce feelings of stress in counsellors.

The presence of secrecy-related problems might be viewed as an opportunity for making overt significant issues which are otherwise difficult to face. The effect of the management of secrets can itself lead to more open communication, not only between the counsellor and patient but between the patient and the other social contacts which constitute his social group.

ELEVEN

The Worried Well

'That's the reason they're called lessons,' the Gryphon remarked: 'because they lessen from day to day.'

Lewis Carroll

INTRODUCTION

The impact of HIV infection on the population at large has always been difficult to measure, but the problems of the 'worried well' constitute an intractable worry about HIV infection which can become incapacitating for the patient and frustrating for the counsellor. Many counsellors describe an impasse in their management of these patients. We have found that counselling so-called worried well patients has challenged our clinical practice, particularly our understanding of and response to *resistance* in counselling and psychotherapy. This chapter defines this patient sub-group and presents some ideas and skills for responding therapeutically to an impasse where resistance to change becomes the main problem in counselling sessions.

WHO ARE THE WORRIED WELL?

The worried well are those who perceive themselves to have been at risk for HIV. They may fear that they have either been infected with HIV or that they already have signs and symptoms of HIV disease, *while in fact they have not been infected.* The presentation of the worried well can be broken into a number of sub-groups.

Those with a previous sex or drug-use history

People who have had unprotected sexual relationships in the past or who have shared needles when injecting drugs, putting them at some risk for HIV, may present as the worried well. Increased awareness of the main routes of transmission of HIV, through government health education programmes, has aroused worries in such people, a proportion of whom may be at risk for HIV.

Those with relationship problems

Fear of HIV infection can indicate difficulties in a person who has problems in entering into, remaining in, and ending relationships. An intractable worry about HIV may signal a call for professional help in a troubled relationship (Salt *et al*, 1989). In this case, the worry is a symptom that helps to regulate the social and emotional distance in the relationship. A fear of HIV may be a convenient excuse for not going out to meet people.

The partners and spouse of those at risk

Another group is the partners of people who have been at risk for HIV. Sometimes a spouse or partner will seek counselling. It may become evident that the worry is for the partner whom the patient suspects may be having an affair outside their relationship. A worry about HIV invariably has an impact on relationships.

Couples in individual and family life-cycle transitions

Couples who are contemplating marriage and people who are going through life-stage transitions within their own family or relationships may present either with HIV-related worries or directly for an HIV antibody test. Points of transition in individual and family life-cycles may exacerbate existing stresses and problems in relationships, leading to additional fears about HIV. This group especially includes parents of adolescents, couples facing the 'empty nest' or who are experiencing a mid-life crisis, people who have been recently bereaved and for whom issues about death and loss seem uppermost in their minds, and individuals who have recently divorced or separated.

Past history of psychological problems

Patients who have a history of psychological problems such as anxiety and depression may also present as the worried well. A worry about HIV may be either a further manifestation of psychological problems or a convenient symptom because themes relating to sex, relationships, dying and care will probably be addressed in counselling sessions. Ex-psychiatric patients who have been discharged back into the community may be represented among this sub-group. Some of these patients may be using HIV counselling facilities as a way of engaging care and counselling as a way into the health care system. Some of the patients may have been at risk for HIV through sex and drug-related activities.

Misunderstanding of health education material

There is a small but important sub-group of people who present for counselling who may have misunderstood statements about safer sex or other means of avoiding HIV infection. Public health eduction in the form of television and media campaigns can only convey limited information. People then need to have a personal interview with someone who has experience in the field for their specific questions and anxieties to be addressed. For a few, misunderstandings of public information remain firmly held.

Pseudo and factitious AIDS

Lastly, there is that group of patients who present either with 'pseudo AIDS' or 'factitious AIDS'. These are both relatively uncommon but interesting presentations of the worried well. The patient believes that he has full-blown AIDS. A number of symptoms may support this, such as diarrhoea, weight-loss and night sweats. Those with 'factitious AIDS' will present in hospital departments saying that they have been tested for HIV, that their result was positive and that they would like to be linked in for medical surveillance and social care. A patient with 'pseudo-AIDS' *fears* being infected with HIV and becoming ill; the anxiety leads to the somatic symptoms which may be interpreted as signs of AIDS by the patient, thus feeding into a spiral of fear. Patients with factitious AIDS, on the other hand, experience some benefit in being defined as ill, being clinically investigated and treated. They may feign AIDS symptoms in order to gain attention.

MANAGING THE WORRIED WELL

Redefinition

The 'worried well' is not an accurate or useful definition for many of these patients. Nobody can be defined as *well* until a doctor has examined and investigated him. Only by a process of exclusion can he be called 'worried *and* well'. For this reason, a patient who presents to a physician or HIV counsellor with an HIV-related worry should be considered as being at risk for HIV until proved otherwise. It is only through history-taking, examination, and testing that the potential for being infected with HIV can be firmly discounted. The difficulty of classifying this condition can pose dilemmas for the physician and counsellor.

Dilemmas

There are a number of dilemmas that counsellors face in counselling the worried well. These may include: (a) whether to test the patient for HIV; (b) whether to refer the patient to a psychiatrist or psychologist; (c) whether or not the patient's general practitioner should be involved so that he can share the care of the patient; (d) whether to reassure a patient without testing him; (e) how to interpret AIDS-like symptoms which may be either a manifestation of anxiety or of HIV disease itself; and (f) how to encourage a patient to bring in a sexual partner for counselling, without breaching confidentiality. Dealing with the worried well is not always a straightforward task. Some patients may implicitly or explicitly say to the physician: 'Tell me that I do not have AIDS, but do not test me for it.' There are a number of procedures and skills which the counsellor should employ with patients who are worried about HIV, but who are otherwise well.

Recognition

There is a range of behaviours and symptoms which indicate that somebody may have a worry about HIV. Often patients do not explicitly voice their worry, instead exhibiting symptoms which hint at their state of mind. The counsellor needs to be experienced to interpret the patient's signals. The patient may exhibit his condition through persistent health checks, anxieties about relationships, worries about sexual dysfunction, panic attacks, and symptoms similar to AIDS. Other patients are more explicit about their worries, and ask for 'an AIDS test', HIV counselling or for literature about HIV. The worry may not always be claimed for the person who presents: he may attribute symptoms to a colleague, friend, relative or another member of the family.

It may be appropriate to discuss directly the worry about HIV and any reported symptoms from the outset. This conveys the message to the patient that HIV concerns can be raised without the need for vague hints or descriptions of a worry in a relative. This approach alone may be sufficient to end some patients' worry and will treat the symptomatic behaviour.

There is a secondary concern for some worried well patients: with whom can they discuss their worry? As a consequence of social stigma and fearing a breach of confidentiality, some patients may not wish to consult their general practitioner or discuss their worries with their family or partner. Many patients have close or longstanding family relationships with their general practitioner. Some may not have told their doctor that they are homosexual, while others may not wish their partner to know of a past sexual liaison. The anxiety symptom may be exacerbated as a result of this self-imposed secrecy.

The start of counselling

There are a number of different strategies for counselling worried well patients. The following guidelines provide a useful framework, although there can be many variations.

1 Ask the patient what it was that made him decide to come to see you. If HIV is not mentioned, but perhaps hinted at, ask if HIV is one of his worries. Assess his knowledge of the facts about HIV and provide information where necessary.
2 Identify what activities the patient thinks have put him at risk for HIV. Discuss unprotected sex, sharing needles in intravenous drug use and

blood transfusion history, if appropriate. Try to understand why the patient has come at this particular point with his worry. Identify individual, family or work stresses or life-cycle transitions. Ask the patient what he thinks would best help him to get over his worry. Offer an HIV antibody test, if appropriate. (For a more extensive discussion about counselling for an HIV antibody test, see Chapter 7.)

3 Ask the patient if he will be reassured by a negative HIV antibody result. If the patient says that a negative result will not be reassuring, ask what would help him to overcome his fear and belief that he has HIV. Refer the patient for testing, further counselling or to a voluntary HIV organization. Offer a follow-up appointment, if this is indicated.

When counselling these patients, find out what they have done about their worries so far. It may be that they have had tests elsewhere, or they may have had to keep their worry about HIV a secret, which has served to exacerbate their anxiety. It may be helpful for the counsellor to ask patients to guide him in how best to help them with their worry. Some say: 'I have been thinking about having a test.' Others say: 'Perhaps I need to see a therapist', and so on.

When relationship problems are suspected, it may be easier to discuss these initially rather than exploring the individual's specific worry. A useful question is always: 'Who else knows that you have this worry?' The answer will give some idea about the patient's support network, whether or not he is keeping secrets from others and how he has dealt with his worry about HIV up to this point.

MANAGING RESISTANCE AND AN IMPASSE IN COUNSELLING

At the stage where the counsellor feels that no further progress is being made in helping the patient to resolve his fear about HIV, innovative therapeutic approaches are called for. An impasse is marked by a 'more-of-the-same' situation (Watzlawick, Weakland and Fisch, 1974) in which any intervention by the counsellor results in 'no change' in the patient system. In counselling the worried

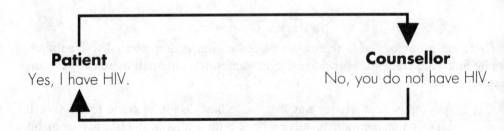

Patient
Yes, I have HIV.

Counsellor
No, you do not have HIV.

well, the symmetrical relationship between the counsellor and patient may be characterized by an increasingly desperate or authoritative counsellor trying to convince an equally rigid patient that he is not infected with HIV, but to no avail.

This can become a game without end and is depicted in the diagram.

There may be variations of this 'game' where the patient fears that he has HIV, but is too frightened to have a test, and the counsellor either reassures the patient or tempts him to have a test, just to prove that the result will be negative. The interaction becomes repetitive and rigid. The following are five examples of these injunctions.

> Test me for HIV; but don't tell me if the result is positive.
>
> If I'm positive for HIV, I will kill myself.
>
> I know this is my fifth visit to discuss my AIDS worry, but I am not having a test.
>
> There must be a mistake. I don't believe the result is negative.
>
> It's my husband. I won't sleep with him until you've tested him.

Traditional theories about resistance in counselling tend to blame the patient for the impasse. In practice, the counsellor may indicate what he perceives as the patient's resistance; or he may slightly vary his interactive behaviour, for example, by raising his voice or adopting a tone of greater authority. The view that we take about resistance is derived from Kelly's (1969) work in psychotherapy. He suggests that the impasse between the counsellor and patient reflects the 'stuckness' of the counsellor rather than the obduracy of the patient. Consequently, the counsellor needs to become more creative in his problem-solving, rather than blaming the patient.

The level of rigidity which characterizes the examples of therapeutic impasse listed above should signal to the counsellor that psychological problems are of greater importance than medical problems. We hypothesize that many of these problems reflect relationship difficulties. Some patients are psychologically fragile and the intense and rigid worry may prevent them from 'cracking up' and developing acute psychiatric problems. A few patients are lonely, and counselling is a relationship for them. For this reason, we emphasize using psychotherapeutic techniques to overcome the impasse, otherwise psychological problems may seriously interfere with the patient's care and management. The counsellor's task at this point is to break the cycle of 'Yes, I am . . . No, you're not' in the first instance. Some of the following strategies may be used to do this:

1   *Comment on the apparent stuckness*
I feel that each time I try to persuade you that you cannot possibly be infected with HIV, you seem to be quite convinced that you are. If you were the counsellor in my position, what might you say to a patient?

2   *Adopt a 'one-down' position with the patient and declare your lack of ideas to help him. (Somewhat theatrically, looking exasperated, hand on forehead)*
Well, well, well; Steven, you seem to have got me here; I just can't think how I'm going to change your ideas. I just don't seem to be able to throw any light on this. I'll need to think about this for a while. Give me a few minutes, please. Why don't you wait outside the office and I'll call you back in a while.

3   *Solicit the patient's help*
Do you have any ideas about what may help to convince you that you don't have HIV? What will reassure you?

4   *Discuss the effect of the worry on relationships*
How has this worry affected your relationship with your children?

5   *Ask what would happen if the worry persisted*
Vanessa, if this worry about HIV never went away, how would you see yourself managing in the future?

6   *Ask what might replace this worry*
If, for some reason, you stopped worrying about HIV, is there anything else you might start to worry about?

7   *Talk hypothetically about living with HIV*
You keep trying to convince me that you have got HIV. You don't believe me when I say the seven tests that you have had were accurate and reliable. Let's pretend for a few minutes that you *do* have HIV. Let's talk about a day in the life of Eric with HIV. How much of the day would you think about HIV? Who would you talk to about it? What would you be doing that is different from what you are doing today? What would be similar?

8   *Discuss some advantages of worrying*
Has your worrying resulted in anything good for you? Think very carefully before you answer.

9   *Convey the idea of a psychological symptom*
In our experience, a worry about HIV can reflect unhappiness or difficulties in other areas of people's lives. Is there anything else happening in your life that you think we should be aware of?

10   *Refer the patient to a psychologist or psychiatrist*
Maybe the time has come to refer you to a specialist for an opinion.

The drive for help

There is a small group of patients who present with HIV-related worries but cannot be reassured by tests, counselling or literature about HIV. This group may keep producing a worry about HIV in order to maintain access to and contact with the counsellor. In such cases, the worry is a ticket of entry to psychological support systems. Unless the counsellor notes this, the patient will revert to the HIV worry at the end of counselling sessions in order to re-engage the counsellor. It can be of some help in these circumstances to say to the patient: 'I will continue to see you for counselling even if you no longer have worries about HIV.' The main concern behind the patient's symptom is then suggested and other issues can be explored.

CONCLUSION

Counsellors need to be sensitive to the different concerns of patients and the indirect ways in which patients may sometimes express these concerns. Therapeutic work with the worried well is among the most complex that counsellors face in HIV management. In some situations, a referral to a psychiatrist or psychologist may be appropriate if the patient's main underlying problem is behavioural and emotional rather than medical. The principles of managing resistance can be applied to other clinical situations in which an impasse develops between the counsellor and patient.

TWELVE

Counselling Women About HIV-related Problems

Conversation is a game of circles. In conversation we pluck up the termini which bound the common of silence on every side.

Ralph Waldo Emerson

INTRODUCTION

As the incidence of heterosexually acquired HIV infection increases, more women are likely to become infected, and many of these will be of childbearing age. Women are doubly affected by HIV disease (Bradbeer, 1989). They have to cope with not only the medical and social consequences, but also the complex issues surrounding childbearing and motherhood. Ideally the issues surrounding HIV should form an integral part of the discussion about other health-related issues with women who attend clinics for family planning and antenatal care. In some cases, counselling about HIV or fertility may reveal other concerns and give rise to problems similar to those that are found in counselling the worried well (see Chapter 11). This chapter addresses some of the issues for women surrounding HIV screening, childbearing and childrearing and offers some guidelines for counselling. At the same time we recognize that some women do not want to have children.

SCREENING WOMEN FOR HIV IN ANTENATAL CARE

Why screen women for HIV?

Unless HIV testing is made easily available to women and becomes accepted as a routine antenatal screening test, like those for syphilis and rubella antibodies, HIV infection may continue to go largely undetected in this population. Some women, unaware that they have been at risk, are infected with HIV. Those women who are aware of their HIV diagnosis may have to make decisions about having children. A decision not to conceive, or failure to conceive, can affect their relationships. Counselling before and after decisions about testing and conception can help women to address some of these problems. HIV screening is important in order to:

- provide women with information on which to make informed decisions about sexual relationships and pregnancy (Black and Levy, 1988);
- offer medical care and treatment to HIV-infected women;
- gather epidemiological data so that adequate and appropriate services can be provided for women and their children. These may include obstetric and gynaecological care and treatment, and facilities for child care;
- reduce the stigma attached to HIV by making the availability of the HIV test, treatment and care more routine and acceptable as is the case for many other diseases.

Who should be screened for HIV infection?

Screening for HIV infection can be either selective or systematic. *Selective screening* involves explaining to the patient what constitutes a risk and asking her to consider being tested. The danger of screening 'at-risk' women is that assumptions may be made about who is infected. Some women, who know that they have been at risk for HIV, may not disclose this to their doctor, while others might have been put at risk without being aware of it (Barbacci *et al.*, 1990).

Systematic screening of all pregnant women at their first antenatal appointment can be carried out in two ways. Either an HIV test can be offered to all women attending the clinic, or all women can be informed that they will be HIV tested, unless they say that they do not wish to be tested. Whichever method of screening is adopted, counselling should be available before the test and when giving results. There should be a multidisciplinary team comprising doctors, nurses and specialist counsellors in place for follow-up care.

Why counsel for screening?

As with any HIV test, counselling should accompany screening for HIV so that women can be prepared for the HIV test and its possible outcome. Counselling provides an opportunity to inform patients about HIV and enables them to make informed decisions about testing, pregnancy, medical care and relationships. It is ethically unacceptable, at present, to carry out an HIV test without the knowledge and informed consent of the woman, and it may compound problems if a positive result has to be given to a pregnant woman who has not been prepared for the test.

GUIDELINES FOR COUNSELLING FOR HIV SCREENING

The guidelines for pre-HIV test counselling for women are identical in every respect to those which have been described in Chapter 7. In addition, some specific issues relevant only to those attending the antenatal clinic are discussed below.

Introduce the HIV test

The counsellor should introduce the HIV antibody test by making it seem a normal and commonplace procedure. An example of a question to introduce the topic for discussion is:

> Among other tests, we offer the HIV antibody test to all expectant mothers who attend this clinic. Have you ever thought about having this test, or had one before?

In order to introduce the idea that anyone might be at risk for HIV, some of the following questions may be asked before discussing any specific risk for the woman:

> Do you know why we offer the test to all women?
>
> What do you know about the risks of passing the virus from a mother to her child at the time of conception, during pregnancy, at the time of delivery and through breast-feeding?
>
> Do you think that you have been at risk for HIV at any time?

Consider the 'window period'

Discussion of the window period between exposure to HIV and the appearance of antibodies is particularly relevant if the woman is at an early stage of pregnancy. She might wish to consider termination if found to be HIV-positive.

> When do you think was the last occasion when you might have been at risk of infection?
>
> If your risk has been within the last three months, would you be prepared to be tested again in a few weeks?

Advantages and disadvantages of HIV testing

The woman must be given the opportunity of considering the advantages and disadvantages of HIV testing for her before making a decision. An HIV test, done as a part of routine screening, does not carry an automatic penalty for life insurance if it gives a negative result.

Decisions about childbearing

Pregnant women being screened for HIV must be counselled to consider the implications of a positive result and how they might react. Some examples of questions are:

> If you decide to have the test, how might a positive result affect your view of

pregnancy? Would you want to continue with the pregnancy or discuss the possibility of termination of the pregnancy?

How would it affect your relationship with your partner if you decided to have a termination?

Informing others

Whereas not all people who come for an HIV test may be in a relationship, a pregnant woman is more likely to have a current partner whose views about the test will need to be considered. Differing views will affect their relationship.

If your partner knew you were considering having the test, what might his views be?

Adequacy of counselling

The woman will need to decide, after counselling, whether or not to have the test. In general practitioners' surgeries or antenatal clinics there may be a greater pressure on time than in other settings where HIV pre-test counselling takes place. A referral to a specialist HIV counsellor might be indicated in some instances.

COPING WITH THE DIAGNOSIS AND PROGRESS OF THE DISEASE

The problems of coping with the diagnosis of a progressive illness have already been discussed in Chapters 8, 9 and 15. Support and advice can be given through counselling and this may help to alleviate some of the psychological and practical repercussions of a positive test result. For women, there are unique difficulties which relate to childbearing and childrearing (Johnson, 1989).

Childbearing

Many HIV-infected women need to make decisions about whether to have children (Novick and Rubinstein, 1987). There may be a possible conflict between the rights and wishes of the woman and the ultimate rights and welfare of the child who may be born, and any other child who may be affected by the birth. If a mother has an HIV-infected child, this child will require attention and her other children may be deprived of adequate care.

Some women initially present at infertility clinics having been unable to conceive. During the course of investigations they are found to be infected with HIV. All HIV-infected women for whom childbearing is an issue should be offered counselling. Those who are unable or unwilling to have children should be offered counselling about this loss for themselves and their partners.

The loss of a choice about having a child can be accompanied by similar feelings to those experienced when there has been a bereavement (see Chapter 16). Some women may decide that they could not risk passing on HIV infection to their child. Others feel that they do not wish to become parents knowing that in the future their own health may deteriorate. These decisions may be influenced by a possible 'loss of face', particularly in cultures where women derive status from having children. Where the expectation and hope of becoming parents has been removed, couples may feel that they have lost their investment in the future.

Childbearing may force HIV into the open if one or both partners are infected with HIV. The future of the relationship may be changed by a decision to have or not to have a child. Fear of transmitting the virus or being infected may introduce additional tensions into the relationship of the couple. It may be difficult for health care workers to avoid disclosing their views about the morality of HIV-infected women having children. Nevertheless, the rights of others to make their own choices must be respected. Those at the 'sharp end', including obstetricians, gynaecologists and midwives, may have special concerns about personal safety in the course of surgery and delivery which could influence the type of intervention they would feel able to offer.

The following examples of questions illustrate some approaches to counselling women or couples about having children.

THE PLACE OF CHILDREN IN A RELATIONSHIP

At what stage in your relationship did you plan to have a child?

What would a child mean to you as a couple?

How would things be different or the same for you with a child?

Who spoke about having a child first?

Which of the two of you wants a child most?

Which of the two of you would be more disappointed if you decided not to have a child?

You appear to have different views about having a child. How do you come to a decision at other times in your life when you have different viewpoints?

THE EFFECT OF HAVING AN HIV-INFECTED CHILD

Since babies inherit their mother's antibodies, you would not know for the first year whether your child was infected. How would you cope with this uncertainty? Who would help you with this?

What problems might you expect to occur if your child had HIV?

If your child became ill who might you turn to for help?

If you and your child were both ill how would you cope?

How might your partner cope?

How might having a child with HIV affect your relationship with your partner and your family?

COPING WITH NOT HAVING A CHILD

The following questions can be used to open discussion and help couples to consider the more distant consequences of having and not having children:

What might it mean to you if you did not have a child?

If for any reason you were unable to have a child, how might it affect each of you? And your relationship?

What would help to keep the relationship going?

What might be some of the sources of stress or conflict?

What would you need to do to show people that you are a still a couple?

How would you respond to friends or family who might question you about being childless?

There are always some risks in either having a child or not having a child. What do you think these are for you?

At what stage would you consider giving up trying to have a child?

What would you have to give up if you had a child?

If you do not have a child, what would this allow you to do instead?

CASE EXAMPLE H: Having children where one of the partners is HIV-positive

Mr A, aged 35, has haemophilia and knows that he has been HIV-antibody-positive for the past eight years. He has come to the clinic with his wife to discuss their wish to have a child, as his wife is now 34. Mr A was also p24-antigen-positive, which suggests a higher degree of infectivity and a poorer prognosis (Eyster *et al.*, 1989).

Mr A:	We want to talk about having a child, as it has been on our minds lately.
Counsellor:	What has made you think about this now?
Mr A:	My wife has been getting upset.
Counsellor:	Mrs A, do you agree with your husband. Is it something that has been upsetting you?
Mrs A:	Yes, I agree, but it is difficult to talk about.
Counsellor:	Is it also difficult for you, Mr A?
Mr A:	Yes, I suppose it's the HIV. I feel bad about it.
Counsellor:	Mrs A, did you know that your husband feels bad about the HIV?
Mrs A:	We never talk about it, but I do want a child.
Counsellor:	Which of you wants a child more?
Mr A:	My wife more than I.
Counsellor:	Are there any issues apart from HIV that might influence your decisions to have a child?
Mr A:	Yes, we have not really enough room in our flat and my wife has a good job at present which I think she would like to keep.
Counsellor:	Mr A, if you were unable to have a child because of HIV how would you see your relationship in the future?
Mr A:	For me it would be the same, but my wife might get very upset. She wants a child.
Counsellor:	Mrs A, what are your views?
Mrs A:	I do want Jack's child. I want something to remember him by if anything should happen to him.

Mr A:	If we don't have a child I would feel guilty, and Jane would be quite in her rights to find someone else.
Counsellor:	Did you know that your husband had this idea?
Mrs A:	I suspected it. We just don't know what to do. I am 34 already and don't have much time.
Counsellor:	What do you know about the risks of passing on HIV to your wife and child?
Mr A:	I know it can happen. It is so hard to decide whether or not to take the risk.
Counsellor:	What would help you with that decision?
Mr A:	If I knew how long I had to live, and if I could be sure that my wife would not get infected.
Counsellor:	None of us knows how long we have to live, but being p24-antigen-positive is thought to increase the risk of transmitting the virus.
Mrs A:	I wish I could have a child for both of us to enjoy, but at the moment I feel I would not be prepared to take the risk of being infected. I have thought about artificial insemination, but we have never talked about it. Perhaps now we can go away and discuss it.

CHILDREARING

Having a child marks a stage of development, individually and for a relationship. For women it also means fulfilling a maternal role. The stage of parenting brings with it different responsibilities. The presence of HIV infection in any member of the family can interfere with and disrupt the developmental cycle through illness and death (Carter and McGoldrick, 1990). In addition, there is the pressure of time on women to have children before they are too old.

Childrearing for HIV-infected mothers is directly affected by whether or not the child is also infected with HIV and whether there are other children in the family (Sherr, 1991).

An HIV-infected woman with an uninfected child

One of the main concerns about the uninfected child of an HIV-infected woman is that the child may become an orphan if both parents are infected and they die. The quality of the relationship between mother and child may be affected by her deteriorating physical and mental health, especially during the child's early developmental years. These children are at risk of orphanhood and abandonment, making early preparation and careful planning of their future an important issue for these women to face, however painful it might be. There is a pressure on the woman and her partner to make plans for their child, particularly if he is also infected.

The dilemma for the mother may be deciding who should be told about her HIV infection, how much should be revealed, and when other family members and people in institutions, such as the school nurses, should be told. An uninfected partner, whether or not he is the father of the child, may have the responsibilities of childrearing if the mother becomes ill, and if she dies. It is increasingly common for grandparents to have to take over a parenting role for their children and grandchildren. If there are no close family ties arrangements have to be made more formally for the future care of the child.

An HIV-infected mother may have to consider what to tell her child about her health as he grows up and reaches a stage of being aware of relationships and family concerns. What the mother might want the child to remember about her can be important for both, and is an area that can be considered in counselling HIV-infected women.

In families where a mother is infected with HIV the family may fear that they will be considered *at greater risk* than others of developing psychological and social problems. Mothers should be helped to make plans for their children. Knowing that she has taken all possible steps to arrange for her children's future will allow her to be more relaxed about dealing with the day-to-day problems of childrearing. This can be regarded as good practice for all parents of children, as nobody's future is ever completely secure.

HIV-infected mother with an HIV-infected child

When both mother and child are infected with HIV, all the above issues are relevant, although there may be the added responsibility for ensuring adequate care arrangements, should both be unwell at the same time. It is likely that an infected child will develop some medical problems quite early in life and the practical and psychological implications of this may be stressful for the mother and others who help and support them. The mother will have a period of increased stress physically and psychologically, and she may neglect her own health if the child becomes ill first. In other circumstances, a mother may be unable to give the child the care that he needs due to her own deteriorating clinical or psychological circumstances. The possibility that neither mother nor child will survive can be very stressful for the immediate family who may themselves require support and counselling.

For families with an infected mother and child the concerns are both practical and emotional. When there is a child with HIV infection, the main issue is whether or not to keep it secret from others inside and outside the family. If it is kept a secret, this may be the beginning of problems that stem from denial of reality, because help and support will almost inevitably be needed at a later point. Unless HIV-infected women are able to share the secret with others invested with the authority and resources for care, adequate plans for future care for themselves and their children will not be made.

Non-infected children of HIV-infected women

The non-infected children of an infected mother may suffer from a lack of attention, particularly if they have an HIV-infected sibling. They may become orphans. The deprivation associated with orphanhood is dealt with differently in various societies and cultures. Where, for instance, whole communities are affected by HIV, this might mean that many children are put into institutions and have to face further deprivation. In certain cases, older children of HIV-infected women may have to become the carers. Traditional generational boundaries become blurred as some children and even grandparents take on parenting roles. A number of children with an infected mother or sibling might not only fear, but also suffer, the consequences of others knowing about HIV. Such children live in the shadow of HIV even though they are not infected. This fear of social stigma is one of the main factors that creates secrecy both within the family and between the family and the outside world.

CASE EXAMPLE I: Decisions about child care for an HIV-infected woman

Sally, aged 30, a single mother, was an injecting drug user and had HIV disease. Her attendance at the hospital for clinical care had been sporadic, and she had not kept appointments in the past. She had been reluctant to spend time discussing her medical or social situation with the counsellor. She had a 3-year-old daughter, Cathy, who had started nursery school. Sally was admitted to hospital with an episode of shingles which necessitated discussion about the care of her daughter during her hospitalization. A neighbour agreed to take care of Cathy for a week. The counsellor felt that the time had come to begin to talk to Sally about the future care of Cathy, should Sally's health deteriorate, and if she were to die. This extract from an interview demonstrates how the counsellor opened the subject of Cathy's care, and helped Sally to think about how she might make plans for Cathy and ease some of her own concerns about the future.

Counsellor:	Sally, for some time I have been wanting to talk to you about what ideas you have about Cathy should you become ill, or should anything happen to you. In order to help you we would like to know what your ideas and plans are, so that we can try to do what you want.
Sally:	I haven't any plans, as I'm quite able to cope now. I find it upsetting to think about it.
Counsellor:	What is it you find upsetting?
Sally:	That I might get sick and who would look after Cathy, and would they look after her as well as I do.
Counsellor:	Do you often think about this?
Sally:	All the time. But I try not to. That is why I come to the hospital as little as possible as it reminds me that I have HIV.
Counsellor:	If you allowed yourself to think about it more, what would you worry about most?
Sally:	Well, actually, how long I've got, and who will be the best person to look after Cathy if I die. I hate talking about this.
Counsellor:	Yes, I can see it is very hard. Have you ever thought that all parents have this to think about as we never know when we might get ill or even have a fatal accident?

Sally:	I hadn't thought of it like that, but I suppose you are right.
Counsellor:	If you were to think about Cathy, who would you ideally want to take care of her if you were not around?
Sally:	My mother, but she is getting a bit old. She knows about the HIV, but not that I used drugs. I avoid talking to her because of that.
Counsellor:	If she was here what do you think she would advise you to do?
Sally:	She would say I should talk to my sister who already has three children, and she might be the best person for Cathy.
Counsellor:	Is there anything stopping you from talking to your sister?
Sally:	I am afraid that if her husband heard about the HIV and the drugs he would shun us.
Counsellor:	Where do you get the idea that he would react like that?
Sally:	He is very conservative, but I'm only guessing. That is what I fear most for Cathy. That she will be shunned.
Counsellor:	Does your sister know that you have this worry?
Sally:	No, I haven't talked to her, but I am sure she would say I'm just being over-sensitive.
Counsellor:	Does your sister know about the HIV?
Sally:	Yes.
Counsellor:	If you were to talk to your sister about Cathy what do you think she would say?
Sally:	I think that she would tell me not to worry and that she would take care of her if anything happened to me.
Counsellor:	If you knew this because you had spoken with your sister, do you think it might make things easier for you in any way?
Sally:	Yes, I would feel more settled.
Counsellor:	I know from what you have said that in fact you have given Cathy's future a lot of thought. You will know, I am sure, when the time is right for you to talk to your sister and mother about the things that are important for you and Cathy.
Sally:	That is right, maybe I will talk to my mother first.
Counsellor:	Even though you may not be ready to talk to your sister or mother, we can talk in the way we have about any concerns in the future.

CONCLUSION

Counselling women about HIV testing and about issues relating to having a child is a cornerstone of their comprehensive health care. The decisions that women have to make are complex and emotive, as are so many other issues in HIV. One of the important tasks in counselling is to help women make informed decisions. Talking about the effect of HIV on a child in the context of family relationships prepares us to think about counselling children with HIV, or those affected by HIV, in the family context. This is discussed in the following chapter. Having children may provide a way of diluting powerful emotions between couples or they can be a conduit for those emotions. When faced with infertility or having to decide against having a child because of HIV, women are reversing a pattern of growth and development in the family life-cycle. This is where counselling approaches that help people to think not only about the losses, but about some of the possible compensations of any situation are important and relevant.

THIRTEEN

Counselling HIV-infected Children and Their Families

'When I use a word,' Humpty Dumpty said, in rather a scornful tone, 'it means just what I choose it to mean – neither more nor less.'
'The question is,' said Alice, 'whether you can make words to mean so many different things.'

Lewis Carroll

INTRODUCTION

Seventy per cent of the children with HIV from European countries who have been reported to the World Health Organization have been infected perinatally; and the incidence in the USA is higher (75 per cent). In developed countries, most perinatal transmissions are associated with an intravenous drug-using parent, but with the increasing heterosexual spread of HIV, many more infected children are likely to be born. Other routes of infection are through transfusion of blood or blood products, unsterile medical equipment or instruments used for ear-piercing, tattooing, scarification or circumcision. Older children may be infected through sexual activity, and in some cases through prostitution. The extent of infection through sexual abuse is unknown. The diagnosis of HIV in a child may be the first indication of HIV in the family, bringing the mother's HIV status into the open and raising questions about the HIV status of her sexual partner.

The emphasis in Chapter 12 was on the hypothetical problems of childrearing which might be faced by women taking the risk of having an HIV-infected child. HIV affects not only the infected child but also the parents, siblings and the extended family. In this chapter we address some of the specific issues facing parents and their children. As children near their teens, the counselling techniques and approaches are increasingly similar to those used for adolescents, as described in Chapter 14.

COUNSELLING FAMILIES WITH HIV-INFECTED CHILDREN

Counselling children is always conducted through the parents or those *in loco parentis*, taking their views into account and respecting their wish to protect their child and rear him in accordance with their beliefs and values. At the same time, counsellors who may also wish to be protective need to learn to accept that it is not possible to protect parents and children from all the pain and grief of chronic illness and death. Their task is to help parents and children find the resources to make coping possible.

The counselling needs of a family change more rapidly than those of any other group, as the family dynamic changes with the age and developmental stage of the parents and children, the progression of HIV disease and the therapeutic advances that are made. As with families where there is no HIV, the shape of the family can change with dissolution and reconstitution of the family group when there is a change in partners. Counselling techniques will also change as access to improved treatment becomes available to more children and results in longer survival. Counselling must be tailored to fit the developmental stage of the child and his family.

Transitional stages are always times of risk to the family and this risk is accentuated by illness. Parents focus on milestones, wondering whether the next transition will be reached. At each stage in normal development, parents are relieved of some responsibility while the child gains more autonomy. In HIV disease, the transitions may be delayed, fixing parents and children in their roles and patterns of interaction for longer. Eventually, transitions may be reversed, with older children needing more rather than less care. Disease progression can result in physical and mental deterioration. For example, opportunistic infections causing diarrhoea may result in a return to nappies long after they have been abandoned. Neurological involvement may be manifested by behavioural problems as well as motor impairment.

When the child has been infected *in utero*, during delivery or through breast-feeding, the prognosis is poor. These children usually have symptoms before the end of the first year of life and become increasingly ill by the second year (Scott *et al.*, 1989). Counselling in these cases must be for the parents and siblings of the affected child, both to help them to cope for themselves, and to find ways of helping the child to deal with illness, painful investigations, hospital visits and admissions.

Parents can be encouraged to think positively about themselves and their ways of coping. If they are enabled to feel that they have gained some control over their lives, they may communicate this feeling of confidence to a child who would otherwise feel threatened by an apparent loss of confidence and authority in an adult on whom he depends.

The problems and counselling approaches for older children infected by routes other than vertical transmission are discussed in detail in the following chapter on adolescents.

COMMON BELIEFS AND VALUES IN FAMILIES

All families have beliefs and values, shaped by their experience of their own families of origin, their culture and their social situation. Some of their common beliefs which may be challenged by HIV are:

Children grow up and leave home, allowing parents to regain their freedom. Children infected with HIV may require increasing rather than decreasing care. Some may never be fit enough to leave home and may in fact not live long enough to achieve other goals.

Children are regarded as an investment in the future. Parents may need to learn to make alternative plans for the future. If infected themselves, they may be unable to fulfil the obligations to their children which they saw as their responsibility. Relatives or representatives of authority may take over their parenting role, or an uninfected parent may become the sole carer. Whether the parent or the child is to be the one to succumb first to HIV, the uncertainty about the length of time they have together can affect the relationship. Decisions about daily living and planning for future care may become difficult.

It is believed that parents must bond with their children. In families where there is a child with HIV, parents must find a balance between becoming totally enmeshed with their child and making too early a separation in anticipation of death, as this may be interpreted as rejection.

The belief is that social service agencies are there to fulfil a supportive role. Some families, where parents' health is in question, may resist social service input. They may regard it as questioning their competence as parents and fear the removal of their children into care by authority care.

Many parents have the belief that they should **sacrifice themselves for their children**, and this may lead them to make unwise gestures, such as giving up work to spend more time with the asymptomatic infected child. On the other hand, when the stage of serious or terminal illness is reached, the parents may need to make sacrifices.

Cultural and religious influences may lead to the belief that **social stigma and ostracism will automatically result from disclosing the diagnosis of HIV**. The resulting secrecy also prevents the sharing of burdens within the family or the extended system, for example, in schools and with friends.

ISSUES TO BE ADDRESSED BY THE COUNSELLOR

Parents

All children born to HIV-positive mothers will have maternal antibodies present from birth, but only about 13 to 39 per cent of these children will actually have been infected with the HIV virus (European Collaborative Study, 1991). The maternal antibodies may take up to 18 months to disappear, so the first uncertainty faced by the parent or parents is whether or not the child has been infected. This uncertainty affects the relationships between parent and child. Parents may become over-anxious and protective, fearing that the child has been infected and anticipating illness. On the other hand, they may resort to denying the risk to their child to avoid confronting the possibility of infection; and in doing this, they may neglect to seek help in time if the child becomes ill.

It is difficult to predict exactly how the disease will progress in children because experience in HIV is limited by the relatively short time since it was recognized, and because new therapies are being developed which may increase the quality of life and length of survival of infected children. Parents must cope with not knowing how long their child has to live and how he may die.

Once it is known that a child is infected, arrangements may need to be made for the care of other children in the family while extra attention is paid to the infected child, particularly if frequent clinic or hospital visits become necessary. There may be financial hardships and housing problems to add to the burden of illness. If one or both parents become ill, care of the children may become increasingly difficult and outside help may become essential – making any secrets difficult to keep. Parents may need to be reminded of the importance of having wills and making provision for fostering and adoption.

The relationship between the parents may deteriorate as a result of the stresses of looking after an ill child with an uncertain future. Either parent may feel that their own emotional needs are not being met by their partner. HIV in the child may lead to a relationship of guilt and blaming for the parents. In the case of a single-parent family the mother may blame herself for passing on the HIV to her child, but in addition may feel resentment and anger towards the partner who infected her and is not there. The need for outside support may be greater for single-parent families. Maintaining an adequate balance between caring for the affected child and keeping life as normal as possible for the rest of the family may be difficult to achieve. The counsellor can help in such situations:

Counsellor: How are you coping with the knowledge that you have a child who might die, and what helps you most to do this?
Mother: We have our religion and that helps a lot now.
Counsellor: If he wasn't here any more how do you see your husband coping?
Mother: That is a good question as I really worry more about him than I worry for myself. I have very strong beliefs that God knows what is right for us.
Counsellor: Who do you think will be able to help your husband most?
Mother: Perhaps me.
Counsellor: In what way?
Mother: By doing more of the things with him that he would like to do.

Parents may have to make decisions about who to tell, how much to tell, how to tell and when to tell about HIV in the family. Some parents may have the view that the child will no longer see a future for himself if the diagnosis is disclosed. There may be fears about confidentiality because the child may be tempted to share the secret outside the family, risking discrimination and stigma for himself and the whole family. The fear of stigma may prevent parents from telling schoolteachers about HIV and thus deprive children, particularly siblings, of the special care and attention they may need to help them cope with illness and possible bereavement in the family. The counsellor can intervene in the following way:

Counsellor: At what age do you think James should be told?

Mrs A: When he's old enough to understand.

Counsellor: What would help you to know that he was old enough to understand?

Mrs A: If he started asking questions.

Counsellor: As he is now eight, what do you think stops him asking questions?

Mrs A: We never talk about it and my husband switches the television off as soon as there is anything about HIV.

Counsellor: In your family, do you ever talk about other things that may seem difficult or do you always wait for questions?

Mrs A: I'm afraid of starting because it might upset him.

Counsellor: Do you think that he might be more upset if he was worrying about his health and didn't know how to tell you?

In the situation where parents are having difficulty with telling the child about their own HIV-positive condition, the following questions may open up helpful discussion:

What makes you so sure Jill has no ideas about HIV?

Do you think discussing HIV openly in the family could help her share any worries she might have?

Could you think of any advantages for you, your wife and your daughter if she knew your diagnosis?

Who might be most relieved if everyone in the family knew?

Siblings

The reaction of children to having siblings with HIV is determined by their age, stage of development and the extent of their knowledge about the health of their infected brother or sister. They may resent receiving less attention than an affected sibling and this can be shown in behaviour changes such as sleep disturbance, depression, hyperactivity, aggression or obsessive behaviours. In addition to the loss they face through the death of a parent or a sibling, they may also have fears about being abandoned or isolated. Parents are able to discuss HIV more easily with their children if there has previously been good communication between them. Discussion is often precipitated by questions from the child after seeing a programme on television or hearing something discussed at school. If parents rehearse how they might answer questions, it is easier for them when the time comes. The following is an example of rehearsing with parents how they might tell a sibling that his younger brother has HIV and may become very ill and die.

John, aged 8, was infected with HIV by a blood transfusion at the age of two. His CD4 count was falling and he was being treated with Zidovudine. His parents were wondering how to tell his 10-year-old sister about his diagnosis before he became very ill:

Counsellor: Mrs S, what do you think Jane needs to know about John?

Mrs S: Well, I suppose that he has AIDS and might die.

Counsellor: How do you think she would react if she knew?

Mrs S: She would be very upset and cry and she might talk to her best friend.

Counsellor: Is there any problem about that?

Mrs S: We live in a small place and we are so worried about other people knowing.

Counsellor: Maybe that is a risk you may have to take to avoid having her feel later on that she was excluded and prevented from sharing something important in the family.

Mrs S: But what will we say?

Counsellor: In our experience it is most helpful to be direct and clear but to do things in stages. You could start by asking her what she thinks is wrong with John.

The infected child

Young children have a short attention span and a limited understanding of the concepts of life, illness and death. For perinatally infected children there may be neurological involvement either directly through HIV or through HIV-related infections (Marcus *et al.*, 1988). Organic damage to the brain slows cognitive development, which may also be affected by the limited interaction with the environment, resulting from motor involvement. A child's failure to reach the expected milestones of development adds to parental anxiety and isolates him from other people. The child may be further isolated by the way in which people recoil from his increasing needs for care and fear the transmission of infection by casual contact with him. The child with chronic illness may perceive his illness as a form of punishment with resultant symptoms of anxiety, depression or withdrawal. Anxiety resulting from repeated clinic or hospital visits which may involve painful investigations may be manifested in a failure to co-operate with carers, for example by spitting out medicine or resisting medical examination. Young children have some concept of separation and loss. As they grow older this experience may be expanded by contact with death through loss of a relative or pet. The child's concept of death and links with AIDS can be explored. For example:

Counsellor: What do you know about AIDS?

Child: You can die from it.

Counsellor: Do you ever think about dying?

Child: I think about what I will look like. Where will I go?

Counsellor: What would you like to look like and where would you like to go?
Child: Mummy says when you die you can be an angel.

Extended family

The extent to which the extended family will be involved with a diagnosis of HIV in one of the family members will depend on how close they have been in the past and how much information has been shared. If a parent as well as a child is infected, family members may perceive themselves as having to assume an unanticipated and possibly unwanted responsibility for the rest of the family. Grandparents may find themselves assuming a parental role again at a time when they may be increasingly dependent on others for care and support. Uncles and aunts may find themselves caring for additional children, and taking them into their own families.

TASKS FOR THE COUNSELLOR

This section deals with the tasks in counselling the parents and their infected child. The wider issues for siblings are discussed in Chapter 14.

Practical concerns, such as housing, finances and transport, must be dealt with in order to free the family to cope with emotional issues. The most important task in trying to address the issues listed above is to help parents and children say things that they might otherwise have difficulty expressing, in an environment where they feel safe. When family members hear each others' worries, it can help them to view their difficulties differently and pave the way for better communication at home.

After finding out how much the parents want their child to know about his medical condition the counsellor can help them to find the balance between disclosing information which is beyond the grasp of the child and keeping secrets which could lead to raised levels of anxiety. Misconceptions can sometimes provoke greater anxiety than the truth. If children discover that their parents have concealed the truth from them, the resulting loss of trust between them may permanently damage their relationship.

The parents need to continue to live from day to day, drawing on their own strengths and identifying the sources of additional help. Children who are old enough to understand can be told about treatment available to keep them well for longer. In the face of life-threatening illness, the family may become paralysed through terror and withdraw from the practical and emotional needs of its members. The task of the counsellor is to reactivate members of the family by helping them to make decisions on a day-to-day basis, drawing on their own strengths and identifying other sources of support. In this way, the family may learn to maintain hope and preserve a sense of competence and control over their lives. For example:

Counsellor: You have missed your last two appointments. Is there anything that makes it difficult to bring Michael to hospital?

Mrs B: You can't do anything. So what point is there in coming?

Counsellor: You are right that there is no cure for HIV, but there are things that can be done to make day-to-day things better for Michael and for all of you.

Mrs B: Like what?

Counsellor: He can be given medicines to prevent some infections and we could offer ideas about transport to hospital and help in the home. Would these help?

Mrs B: In some ways.

COUNSELLING GUIDELINES AND EXAMPLES

Children in the 1990s are growing up with an increased awareness and knowledge of HIV through the media, school and discussions in the home. Their parents may feel reserve about discussing sex openly or they may have experienced the era of greater sexual freedom between the 1960s and 1980s, and so may be able to talk with less inhibitions about sexual matters.

For those children who have reached the stage at which they are curious and ask questions, answers should be direct, clear and restricted to the level of understanding expected at the developmental stage of the child. The topic of HIV is best addressed in general terms before any specific reference is made to the infected family member. Terms that are familiar to the family should be used. At each stage, the child's level of understanding should be checked by asking questions such as:

Do you ever talk about HIV in your family?

Do you know what we are talking about, James?

Some of the following questions can be used to help parents consider when and how to tell children about HIV.

What is your main concern about telling George about his HIV infection?

If he did become very upset how would it show?

How would you respond if he showed signs of being upset?

At what age do you think he would be ready to be told?

How would you know he was ready?

Would you think it was better to tell him while he is well, or when he might become ill?

Do you think that not raising the subject of HIV might prevent him from asking questions?

Who do you think would be most relieved when he is told?

How might talking about the HIV affect the relationship with George?

In order to establish what the parents see as problems for themselves or their children the counsellor could first ask them how they would know if their child was happy, sad or worried. Parents can be asked what they think might be the child's main worry. Discussing this openly may prevent an escalation of the worry. The child could also be asked whether he worries about his mother becoming ill. For example:

Mrs P: James is very quiet lately.
Counsellor: James, your Mum says you're very quiet. What are you thinking about when you are quiet?
James: Nothing.
Counsellor: What does nothing look like?
James: (Smiles and looks at mother)
Counsellor: Mrs P, what do you think James thinks about when he is quiet?
Mrs P: I don't know. He's usually quiet when we have to go to hospital.
James: I hate those injections.
Counsellor: Do you know why you get injections in the hospital?
James: (Silence. Looks at mother) I don't know.
Counsellor: Could you tell James, Mrs P?

The manner of ending such a session is very important as it can help to contain anxieties by recognizing how people are coping, and offering support in the form of future meetings. For example, the counsellor may end the session as follows:

> I have heard today that you, Mrs P, are worried about when to tell James more about his health and yours. Although your husband is not here today you think that he has the same worries but that he tries to ignore them. Maybe in this way he is helping you to live from day to day and deal with problems as they arise.
>
> James, you say that you are worried about needles and injections. We have told you that you need them to try to make your cough better. These are things that you can talk about to us and to your mother.
>
> Mrs P, James has worries that you have heard about for the first time today, but he has been able to tell us and so you will be able to help him when he has more worries. We will meet again the next time you come to the clinic.

CONCLUSION

Counsellors can use the experiences they already have about how to introduce new ideas and subjects, such as sex, to children by taking their lead from the child and only giving information as the child indicates that he understands it. In other words, the counsellor should follow the developmental stages for the particular child. It is also important not to neglect the needs of the uninfected children in the family; their emotional needs may be as great as those of the infected child. There is often a great temptation for the counsellor to take on more responsibilities in the field of HIV than in other work, because there is often loneliness and isolation. Nowhere is this stronger than in working with children and their parents, because of the emotional issues from working with dying children. A counselling approach which returns some responsibility to the family for resolving dilemmas may lessen this danger. Through teamwork, professional supervision and consultation, the counsellor should derive much needed support in working with children and families affected by HIV.

FOURTEEN

The Adolescent and HIV

*The value of life lies not in the length of days but in the use you make
of them.*

Montaigne

INTRODUCTION

For the adolescent, poised between childhood and adulthood, risk-taking and experimentation are normal activities. This may make them as vulnerable as adults to the risks of being infected with HIV through sex or sharing needles in intravenous drug use. Talking convincingly with young people about sex, drugs and HIV, passing on information about viral transmission and addressing the concerns of those already infected, is a major challenge to the counsellor. In this chapter we consider some of the problems which are unique to adolescence, and the counselling approaches which may be used to address them while still adhering to the basic tenets of 'Hypothesizing, circularity, and neutrality' (Cecchin, 1987; Selvini-Palazzoli *et al.*,1980b).

In the 'looking-glass' world of HIV, all is reversed. Young people die, others find themselves caring for very ill parents when they are still young enough to have expected their parents to continue to care for them. Adolescents may be *infected with* or only *affected by* HIV. Experience gained from dealing with HIV-infected patients with haemophilia and their families has helped us to develop some principles and guidelines which may help when counselling this age group.

ADOLESCENTS WHO HAVE BEEN INFECTED WITH HIV

Adolescents who have acquired HIV may have been infected through any of the following routes:

(a) Blood or blood products. For example, haemophiliacs, thalassaemics, and recipients of blood transfusions for other reasons.
(b) Nosocomial infection. For example, through use of unsterile equipment while receiving medical treatment.
(c) Sexual transmission, whether through heterosexual or homosexual relationships, adolescent prostitutes, or sexual abuse.
(d) Sharing intravenous needles during drug use.
(e) Skin-piercing or tattooing with unsterile needles.

Children infected in any of these ways may now survive longer as a result of antiviral and prophylactic antibiotic therapy, so that the number of HIV-infected adolescents in the mid- to late teens is likely to increase at the present time. Children infected vertically from HIV-positive mothers do not survive long enough to reach adolescence.

The *context* in which the adolescent is seen will determine the counselling approach to be used. In the United Kingdom, adolescents remain legally under parental jurisdiction until they are 16 years old. The rights of parents, or those *in loco parentis* must be respected. There may be conflicts between the wishes of parents and adolescents, particularly if there is a desire to keep secrets. An adolescent may request an HIV test without parental knowledge: parents of an infected adolescent may be reluctant to disclose the diagnosis to him.

'Street children', who may have been infected through any of the previously mentioned routes, could have additional problems. Their impoverished social condition might not only directly affect their life expectancy but also mean that there is no relative responsible for them. Consequently, social agencies might have to take responsibility for decisions about their care and treatment, and how these decisions are to be implemented.

Most healthy adolescents do not concern themselves with the problems of acute or chronic illness, and sexually transmitted diseases may not rank high in their concerns for their own well-being. Nevertheless, the risk of HIV infection is increasing in most parts of the world, and there is an urgent need for better health education for children and young adults. Parents may find that HIV compounds the difficulty of discussing sensitive issues such as sex with their children. There is a need to alert a healthy adolescent to the risks of HIV infection, or to warn one who is already infected of the importance of preventing transmission of infection to others.

HIV testing

Tests may be requested by the adolescent or by the medical attendants. For those under the age of 16, permission for testing must also be obtained from the parents or legal guardians. Counselling at the time of an HIV test is as important for adolescents as it is for adults. This may or may not include the parents if the patient is over 16. In the pre-test session a balance must be found between giving adequate information and raising anxiety beyond the level with which the adolescent can cope while waiting for the results. When giving a positive result, it is essential to identify the sources of support for the adolescent. If parents are to be the main providers of support they may need counselling to enable them to cope with their own emotions, thus helping them to be supportive.

Maintaining some hope for the future is a major challenge for parents and health care providers. The risk of suicide cannot be overlooked when breaking bad news to an adolescent, who may act impulsively. Other adolescents may feel cheated by life and seek what they see as 'revenge' through rebellion and risky behaviour. While not concealing the truth from the adolescent, the counsellor must counterbalance the shock following the news of a positive result by giving information that is realistic and hopeful. For instance, practical information on the availability of antiviral treatment and the support systems for patients and families should be given.

CASE EXAMPLE J: Taking small steps to make the future more manageable

When faced with an overwhelming sense of loss of future, identifying small, attainable goals can restore to the patient some feeling of control over his life. The following case example illustrates how some of these ideas were discussed with Robert, a newly diagnosed 15-year-old.

Robert:	What is the point of staying on at school if I'm going to die?
Counsellor:	We don't know when anyone is going to die even if they have AIDS. Supposing you were to live for at least another ten years, what would you want to do with the time?
Robert:	Photography and travel.
Counsellor:	Have you thought about how you might achieve this if you decided to leave school when you are legally able to do so next year?
Robert:	Get a part-time job. I've looked for a job, but there aren't any around.
Counsellor:	Would it make it easier to get a job if you stayed longer at school?
Robert:	Probably, but it takes so long.
Counsellor:	Have you thought about joining the photography society at school so that you don't need to wait so long before starting to do what you want to do?

Some adolescents may not comply with medical treatment and fail to attend for follow-up. Visits to hospitals or clinics may serve as a reminder of their condition and its implications. Their very real but perhaps unexpressed fears need to be addressed early in the course of the disease. If this is not done, such fears may escalate into larger psychological problems that they cannot handle, such as the fear of going mad or being in pain. For example, Robert had confided in one of the nursing staff that he was afraid of dying. The nurse had told him that he would ask the counsellor to talk to him about his fears.

Counsellor:	The nurse has told me that you have talked to him about dying. Is there anything about dying that you would like to talk about today?
Robert:	What is it like?
Counsellor:	Do you mean dying, or being dead?
Robert:	I don't care about being dead; it's dying. Is it painful?
Counsellor:	Some conditions can be painful, but with the things we can do now, it is unlikely and unnecessary for anyone to be left to suffer pain. There are many things available to relieve pain.

Relationships

If there is HIV infection, negotiating and making relationships in adolescence, both within and outside the family, is made more complex. Fears of ostracism, stigma and discrimination may be viewed as deterrents to open communication. For an adolescent, witnessing friends and peers become ill and die could be very frightening and will become increasingly common as more adolescents become infected.

Parents must strike a balance between promoting independence and setting boundaries for their adolescent children. While wishing to escape the limits of authority in order to achieve freedom, fear of the unknown may result in the adolescent wishing for greater boundary setting and resistance from parents. Some HIV-infected adolescents want to abandon ideas of work and school, and may put pressure on parents to allow them to carry out all their wishes with few restrictions. Increasing reliance on others for physical and emotional care and support reverses the usual progression to greater autonomy and can escalate the conflicts between parents and the HIV-infected adolescent. Some parents may respond by becoming over-protective, while others may be tempted to allow their child greater freedom because his life may be short. If the diagnosis has been made before puberty the parents may postpone disclosing the diagnosis until they feel there is a danger that the infection may be passed on through a sexual relationship. Having a secret may add to the tensions in the family, as already discussed. Some HIV-infected parents do not discuss the diagnosis with their adolescent children for fear of the repercussions, involving difficult questions about death or even social isolation by their peers.

Peer pressure to have a sexual relationship and talk about it in a competitive atmosphere places great stress on all adolescents. Those who are infected with HIV may decide to avoid any risk of having a sexual relationship and thus feel isolated. Others may wish to embark on a sexual relationship and the decision raises dilemmas for the HIV-positive adolescent, the sexual partner, the parents of both and the health care providers. The adolescent may consider it unnecessary to disclose his HIV positivity if precautions advised for safer sex are being taken,. He may also keep his diagnosis secret because he fears that disclosure will end the relationship. Parents and health care providers may also have dilemmas about their responsibility to the sexual partner of the adolescent, particularly if there are indications that the diagnosis has not been disclosed.

The counselling of HIV-infected adolescents differs in some ways from counselling adults. There are particular aspects of counselling which are unique to this age group and present a particular challenge. These require tact and sensitivity in order to engage the adolescent's attention sufficiently to enlist his co-operation. Counsellors may thus facilitate conversations between adolescents and their parents or guardians, and ensure that the risks of transmission are fully understood. Parents may wish to have some time to discuss their concerns apart from the family interview which includes the adolescent. Decisions about this should be made after open discussion to avoid suggesting that the counsellor might be viewed as having an alliance with either parents or adolescent.

Counsellors must make clear statements, using language understood by the adolescent. The counsellor should not make assumptions about how much has been understood. He should ask questions to check the extent of the adolescent's knowledge and reinforce the information.

GUIDELINES FOR THE COUNSELLOR

Rapport must be established so as to enable the adolescent to discuss what may seem to be difficult topics. Brief conversations with elements of surprise and some humour may engage the adolescent more easily than long discussions, which often result in a loss of concentration.

Consider how the referral may affect counselling. Although the adolescent will probably have been referred to the counsellor by his parents or other figures in authority, he is likely to be far less resistant if he has asked for help himself.

The adolescent will quite possibly demonstrate feelings of resistance, scepticism and a distrust of counselling. These feelings are appropriate to the situation. He may indicate what he feels by coming late or missing appointments, not taking advice from the counsellor, or through non-verbal behaviours such as chewing gum, not talking or putting his feet on office furniture. The counsellor will be an unwelcome figure for most adolescents. It would probably be strange if this were not the view of these young patients. The counsellor must therefore accept that in many cases he is working with a 'resistant' patient (see Chapter 11).

A further problem for the counsellor is that some HIV-infected adolescents may not have good links with health care agencies since many come from chaotic and deprived social backgrounds. To avoid an argument the counsellor might attempt to deal with resistance by sharing the adolescent's scepticism about counselling, if this becomes an issue, and confirming his views. As in the adolescent's relationships with parents, the counsellor needs to balance this approach with a firmness which conveys boundaries and gives him something to 'push' against. The alternative, in some cases, is for the counsellor to battle on trying to convince the adolescent of his view, incurring a major act of defiance; the adolescent may even opt out of sessions, ending any further influence over him.

One of the aims of counselling an HIV-infected adolescent is to normalize his situation for him, as much as is possible under the circumstances, without denying reality. On the one hand, the counsellor can help him to grow and develop as a person, to experiment, to take some risks, to be rebellious and to have hopes and dreams for his future. On the other hand, the counsellor has to try to help him not to endanger others, for example by infecting them. He should help the adolescent to acquire a modified view of the future and his prospects for relationships. Harm minimization, to himself and others, is a guiding theme for the counsellor. However, it seems improbable and inappropriate that the counsellor will be able to eliminate every risk situation in the adolescent's life.

Some adolescents will view the counsellor as intrusive and meddlesome. We try to convey to our patients that we *cannot instruct* them or make them do anything they do not want to do. As counsellors, we are not agents of social control: we cannot ensure than an HIV-infected adolescent is protecting his sexual partners from infection. Instead, we try to enhance the responsibility of the patient or those in authority, such as the parents.

Social workers or doctors will encounter problems in counselling adolescents who perceive that the counselling process conceals the imposition of unwelcome ideas. However, there will be times when the counsellor feels that legal issues must be at the forefront of discussions with the patient – for example, if he confesses to dealing in drugs (Girardi *et al.*, 1988). At this point, the counsellor must be open and tell the patient that his role has been changed by his legal responsibility to others as well as to the patient. The need to deal with this alters the relationship between the counsellor and patient as they may have to discuss counselling duties, responsibilities and accountability. This new emphasis need not be detrimental to the counselling relationship.

The structure of the session

The counsellor should keep sessions focused and brief, try to engage the adolescent by introducing novelty to his approach (Young and Beier, 1982). The offer of practical help, such as advice about available financial support, and the obtaining and use of condoms, will demonstrate that the counsellor has a wider competence than simply dealing with 'crazy people', which may well be the adolescent's expectation of counselling.

The counsellor should be willing to talk about 'non-HIV matters' such as parent–teenager conflicts, career decisions and emerging sexual relationships. He should also discuss how the adolescent sees his future.

The problems of HIV and haemophilia

There is an added dimension to the dilemmas of children and parents when the adolescent is haemophilic and has been infected by contaminated blood products. Haemophilia is a life-long, incurable disorder kept in check by intravenous infusions of the missing coagulation factor. These necessary infusions which were considered to be a 'life-saver' have, for some, become the destroyer of their future. Mothers may feel guilty because they have not only passed on the haemophilia but, in many cases, have actually unknowingly injected the contaminated product. Many health care workers, who are accustomed to saving lives, feel responsible for having prescribed and administered the factor concentrate.

Some adolescents may feel anger and resentment at having been infected in circumstances beyond their control, with rage and frustration leading them to engage in irresponsible and rebellious behaviour directed against all authority, including parents and health care providers on whom they lay blame for their infection. Others may feel helpless and withdraw into depression and isolation.

These reactions are similar to those of other infected adolescents.

In terms of medical care, haemophilic adolescents have the advantage of being part of a life-long caring system. The haemophilia centres which provide their regular health care can continue, in some contexts, to provide medical, psychological and practical support for the patient and his family.

When the haemophilic adolescent has been infected as a young child, the parents have to decide how, when and who will inform him of his infection. As with other groups of adolescents, many parents postpone this until puberty when, they say, 'sex may come onto the scene'. Some choose to tell the adolescent themselves, others may enlist the presence of health care staff to provide support and answer questions. Parents only rarely leave this task to the counsellor.

Haemophilia has always added to the problems of making relationships. An infected adolescent will now need to find ways of telling a prospective partner about HIV as well as about haemophilia. A counsellor can facilitate this difficult admission by rehearsing with the young person how he might open up discussion about HIV before starting a sexual relationship and offering to see the couple together.

CASE EXAMPLE K: Discussing the effects on an adolescent of having HIV.

A family interview with parents and a boy of 15 with haemophilia and HIV is used to illustrate how concerns are identified and information that might previously have been kept secret is shared with family members. His 13-year-old brother is at school and has not been brought to the interview.

Counsellor:	Mr J, what have you told Peter about why we are here today?
Mr J:	I said we were coming for a check-up and to discuss anything that is worrying us.
Counsellor:	Is this what you understood, Peter?
Peter:	Yeh.
Counsellor:	Mrs J, your husband said you had all come to discuss your worries. Is there anything that you think is worrying your husband?
Mrs J:	Yes, there is. It is what effect it will have on Peter knowing now that he has HIV. We are worried sick.
Counsellor:	What most worries you, Mrs J?
Mrs J:	That he won't be able to marry and have children.
Counsellor:	Peter, did you know that Mum was worried about this?
Peter:	Not really.
Counsellor:	Do you worry about not having children?
Peter:	Not really.
Counsellor:	Peter, I wonder who you think might worry most about this, you, your father, mother, your grandparents or your brother?
Peter:	I don't worry about it. My mother does and so does granny. She only wants me and my brother to have kids.
Counsellor:	So, Peter, you think that granny puts pressure on mother?
Peter:	She is always worrying about those things.
Counsellor:	Mrs J, did you know that Peter thinks you and your mother are most worried about this and Peter least?
Mrs J:	I didn't realize that was how he saw it.
Counsellor:	Mr J, what is your greatest worry today?
Mr J:	That Peter won't work at school because he won't see the point.
Counsellor:	What do you think about what Dad has said?

Peter:	He just worries that we get good jobs. I find work boring at school.
Counsellor:	What would you prefer to be doing?
Peter:	I don't know. There isn't any point, is there, if I'm going to die. You die of AIDS, don't you?
Counsellor:	Yes, you can die of AIDS. Is dying something that worries you?
Peter:	I don't worry about dying. I won't know about anything then. I just want to do what I want.
Counsellor:	What do you want Peter?
Peter:	Not to be nagged all day.
Counsellor:	Just say, Peter, that you keep as well as you are for a good number of years. How would you fill your time?
Peter:	I could get a job.
Counsellor:	Mr J, what is your view about what Peter has been saying? Do any of us know exactly how much time we have got? We could have an accident tomorrow. Do you think that you could discuss with Peter how he might do what he wants, but also show him how difficult it is to get jobs without any qualification? Mrs J, we have heard from Peter that he is not worried about dying. Nor is he worried that he might not marry and have children. He gave me the idea that there are many people who can't have children. Some never find partners, some have other illnesses, and others are infertile. So, although this is your worry now, Peter's worries seem different.

Adolescents affected by HIV

An adolescent may be affected by HIV in the following ways: a parent, sibling or other family member is infected; or a sexual partner is discovered to be HIV-positive. An adolescent may be inhibited from the development of any relationships for fear of the sexual transmission of the disease.

The infected parent has to decide whether the uninfected adolescent should know about his father's or mother's HIV infection while the parent is well and able to discuss plans for the adolescent's future. The alternative is for the parent to wait so long that he is ill and there are indications of approaching death. Counsellors can assist parents in coming to a decision about disclosing their HIV-positive condition by questioning and presenting them with possible alternative scenarios. For example, they might ask:

Would it be at all helpful for your wife if your daughter knew now that you have HIV?

What would be the worst thing that could happen if you told your children about your condition?

Who could help you most in talking with your children about HIV?

HIV can put pressure on the natural ebb and flow of closeness and distance between siblings. The uninfected sibling may experience guilt at being free of the restrictions imposed by infection. An emotional distance may develop in a family between those who know about an HIV diagnosis and those who do not know. Emotional tension may be exhibited by behavioural disturbance such as stealing or school truancy.

Ending the session

How sessions are ended is important, particularly if they have been brief and selective in focusing on subjects for discussion. Arrangements must be made for follow-up. For example:

> I don't know whether you will want to phone me but I would like you to know that this is how you can reach me if you have any questions to ask before we meet again . . ..

CONCLUSION

The most difficult task in counselling adolescents is to address the realities of life-threatening illness for them or for someone close to them, while maintaining some hope. Discussion must be appropriate to the age and stage of development. The adolescent may give the impression of being mature and well-informed, but no assumptions should be made about his ability to understand and assimilate information. As part of normal adolescent rebellion, the adolescent may resist acting on the advice given.

Many parents seek to protect their children from knowing their own diagnosis or that of the other parent or a sibling, because they consider them to be vulnerable and unable to cope with the threats of illness and death. Parents and counsellors must recognize that there are limits to the amount of protection which is beneficial. Failure to talk openly may be more damaging than knowing the truth.

FIFTEEN

Counselling in the Terminal Care Phase of HIV Disease

For just when ideas fail, a word comes in to save the situation.

Goethe

INTRODUCTION

Working in the field of HIV has brought into sharp focus the whole concept of loss, be it psychological or physical. Clinical practice has shown that ideas about, and feelings of, loss may start from the moment a person thinks about HIV in relation to himself or someone else. In some cases, conversations about loss may be introduced from the very first counselling contact, whether it is in a pre-HIV test session or after a diagnosis of HIV infection. This chapter presents some of the ideas and approaches relevant to counselling about loss, whether it relates to terminal illness or bereavement, and introduces some counselling approaches appropriate to the terminal phase of HIV disease.

THEORETICAL IDEAS ABOUT LOSS

There are several theories about the psychological aspects of death and dying which help in the formulation of a clinical approach to loss and bereavement (Kubler-Ross, 1970). Recently, this approach has also been discussed in relation to the field of HIV disease (Green and Sherr, 1989). Views about bereavement and approaches to counselling the bereaved may be related to a theoretical understanding of change and loss in relationships (Carter and McGoldrick, 1989). As a function of emotional growth and development, individuals are constantly undergoing changes in their relationships. Death and dying are a point on the arc of the wider life-cycle, which in the context of the family and social relationships, and belief systems, continues after death. Terminally ill patients have to find ways of coping with these life-cycle changes. Problems may occur if they do not adjust and cope effectively with these changes.

THEORETICAL IDEAS ABOUT COUNSELLING THE TERMINALLY ILL

Ideas about loss and dying may be introduced at an early stage of HIV counselling. This early counselling is a way of preparing people for dealing with actual loss if this does occur (see Chapter 5). Initially, the counselling may be around the loss of health or the cessation of full and active participation in daily life and relationships. As the disease progresses, the patient may experience additional losses, for example, loss of eyesight or ability to work, and the counselling must adapt to this worsening condition. Ideally, the initial counselling will have laid some of the groundwork for further discussions and this may help the patient to deal with these losses.

Reactions to loss may include feelings of grief and sadness expressed by crying, or even a desire to be left alone. These are not the only responses, and, while still grieving, some people may even experience some relief when death finally occurs and ends the patient's suffering. Although death may bring an end to the suffering of patients and their close contacts, it may also simultaneously create new problems. The death of a patient with HIV may be the beginning of a variety of new problems for close contacts of that person. Sexual partners, for example, may also have been infected and will think about their own problems for the first time. In some instances, the AIDS diagnosis of a child may have been the first indication that there is HIV in the family. The new problem that may arise after the patient dies is that attention shifts to the health and future of a surviving partner or family member. Loss, of course, may be complicated by the social stigma and fear of HIV transmission when the cause of death is revealed.

Time and timing are important aspects of the counselling process. Friends and relatives and health care providers may sometimes complicate reactions to loss and bereavement by 'pushing' someone to confront his loss at a time when he is not ready to do this. An accurate assessment of the stage which patients with HIV or the bereaved have reached will contribute significantly to more effective counselling by ensuring that the counsellor is at the 'same place in time' as his patient.

WHAT ARE SOME OF THE LOSSES IN HIV?

There may be multiple physical, mental, economic and social losses resulting from HIV infection at the different stages of infection and illness. These losses could include poor health, a deterioration in the ability to concentrate, memory impairment, and loss of mobility, of dexterity, and – in economic terms – of employment, finances and housing. There may be diminished freedom of choice in many aspects of life, such as international travel or employment.

Although there might be a special emphasis on counselling the dying patient and the bereaved, this is but one aspect of the counsellor's activity.

Counselling issues in the terminal care phase

During the terminal care phase of HIV disease, management and psychological issues may influence how health care providers counsel patients and their contacts. These include dealing with confidentiality and secrets; organizing and settling legal and financial affairs; resolving relationship difficulties; dealing with dependency; talking about and coming to terms with dying; exploring feelings of hope and hopelessness and ending relationships.

Confidentiality and secrets

Although issues of confidentiality require attention at all stages of HIV disease, they become more complex and pressing in the terminal care phase of illness. Chief of these is the question of who should know about the diagnosis and the changing medical condition which inevitably arises. Such problems are less likely to interfere with the patient's management if they have been discussed with him before his deteriorating condition necessitates admission to hospital. Patients' views about who should be kept informed of their condition should be recorded in the medical and nursing notes. It is important that the patient's views are checked from time to time in case they have changed.

Counsellors often find that they become very much more involved with the patient's family and friends at the terminal stage of illness. As the time of death approaches, they may seek information, reassurance, comfort or simply contact at a time when their own social support system may be taxed or withdrawn. In some cases, relatives may try to engage the support of those who are involved with the care of the patient by frequent complaints or arguments. This is often a way of venting feelings difficult to show within the family, and the counsellor may feel the burden of this behaviour.

In addition, a patient may want his relatives to receive counselling to relieve him of the burden and strain of having to give them emotional support. This raises questions about confidentiality and secrets, particularly if the relatives are aware that the patient is terminally ill but do not know about the HIV. The extent of their knowledge must be clarified between the counsellor and patient before any relatives are seen. In some cases, we have found that relatives and close contacts seek help from the patient's counsellor without the knowledge of the patient. It must be made clear to the relatives that, in such instances, the discussion will be limited to concerns or difficulties that *they may have* in relation to the patient's illness. Personal details about the patient will not be revealed unless the patient's permission is obtained. For example:

Counsellor: Does your brother know that you have asked to see me?
Brother: No. I wouldn't want him to know.
Counsellor: If he did know, how do you think he might react?
Brother: I'm not sure, he might be pleased.
Counsellor: What might he be pleased about?

Brother: Well, it might be of some relief to him that I have someone to talk to about my worries.

Counsellor: I am happy to talk to you about your worries, but as with any other patient, I cannot give you any information about his condition as we do not have his permission.

Many counsellors will be familiar with situations where there is pre-existing conflict between family members and the partner of the patient which emerge in the terminal care phase of illness. Counsellors sometimes find that they have to deal with conflicts about keeping the diagnosis secret or taking responsibility for important decisions. Ideally, such difficulties should be pre-empted much earlier in discussions with the patient about how professional carers should best respond to these situations. An extract from an interview with a patient and his boyfriend illustrates how this may be approached:

Counsellor: What does your mother know about your relationship with Tim?
Patient: She thinks that he is just a friend. I've never told her more.
Counsellor: Would you now like her to know more?
Patient: Yes, because they may meet.
Counsellor: If your mother meets Tim and she asks him about your diagnosis, do you think he would tell her?
Patient: If he is stressed he might just 'blow it'. I think he feels angry that I won't tell her about us.
Counsellor: How do you think your mother would react if she did know about your relationship with Tim?
Patient: I don't know, but I think it may be better for all of us.
Counsellor: Does Tim know this?
Patient: No.
Counsellor: What stops you from talking to Tim about this?
Patient: Once I talk to him I may not be able to avoid telling her and I am afraid that she may reject him.

Organizing and settling legal and financial matters

Making a will is a practical step that, in a concrete way, acknowledges the possibility of death. Experience suggests that a will is better made when people are well. However, the task of making a will is neither routine nor familiar for young people and they may need help. Opportunities should be made for the patient to consider the benefits of making a will and the implications of not making a will before he becomes too ill to make his own decisions. The act of contemplating a will, or indeed writing it, may prompt some people to think more about dying, and the psychological benefits of 'getting one's affairs in order' should not be overlooked. An extract of a conversation between a counsellor and a patient about making a will illustrates this:

Counsellor: Paul, have you ever thought about making a will?

Patient: No. It is too much to think about with everything else.

Counsellor: Is there anything that might be made easier for you if you were to decide to think about making a will?

Patient: I'm not sure. I might feel a bit more settled.

Counsellor: More settled in what way?

Patient: Well, I'd know my girlfriend would be taken care of, and I could also say exactly what things I would want my mother to have.

By neglecting to make a will some patients may indirectly communicate that they prefer others to make decisions for them about their estate, and consequently about their relationships. Once a patient has been given opportunities to consider the implications of making a will he should be left to decide, in his own time, what he wants to do. He might then feel that he wants to talk about the implications of not making a will. These are examples of some of the questions that could be asked:

> Do you know what would happen to your boyfriend if you were to die without making a will?

> What ideas might your partner have if she knew that you had not made a will and all your possessions were to go automatically to your family?

> What message would it convey to your boyfriend about your relationship with him if you do not make a will?

There are other practical steps that a counsellor might need to take in order to help a patient feel more settled about the future. These include the clarification and assessment of financial and social support, and an examination of the available options for care he would choose, if, for example, he lost his eyesight, ability to make decisions, or became physically dependent. Counsellors may arrange for the patient to obtain advice from legal or financial advisers. Most patients with HIV have worries similar to these (see Chapter 5).

Counsellor: Paul, you say that you have so many worries about the future. What are these?

Paul: We have talked about the stress of my boyfriend if I become ill, and I have decided to see a lawyer about making a will. But that is only one thing. I am worried about what happens if I get too ill to work. How would I manage without money? It is all very well to talk about wills!

Counsellor: There are a number of state benefits that can be claimed. Have you got any insurance policies that might be of use?

Paul: I do have a good accountant and I think I should talk to him. Can you tell me about the state benefits?

Resolution of past relationship conflicts and difficulties

It is sometimes assumed that it is imperative for the family and other close contacts to resolve past conflicts or settle 'unfinished business' between them before someone in the family dies. Whilst it may be appropriate to facilitate this process, it is equally important to assess when *not* to pursue these ends and, if necessary, to help people adjust to and cope with 'unfinished business'. The following dialogue illustrates how the counsellor can help family to leave some business unsettled:

Sister: I read a book once which said that secrets between people are harmful. But my brother and I worry that if he is open about his drug problem, it would upset my parents so much that they would abandon David.

Counsellor: Are you both happy to keep this secret from them?

Sister: As happy as one can be in keeping a secret from one's parents.

Counsellor: What are you both open about with your parents?

Sister: Everything else. They know he's ill, they know it's AIDS, and they're OK about thinking that it came from an ex-girlfriend of David's. It would be awful for all of us if my parents got very upset about drugs.

Counsellor: What will help you to keep this secret?

Sister: It won't be easy not to just let it slip out, but we will have to watch out not to. Maybe we can tell them after he dies.

Dependency

When a patient is very ill or dying, dependency on others can result in a loss of dignity. The patient may become completely dependent on others for basic hygiene activities – for example going to the toilet, bathing and brushing teeth. If he is bedridden, then he may rely on others for most activities such as preparing food. In hospital it is usually nurses who take on some of these intimate tasks. Reassuring statements to the patient, which do not ignore the embarrassment of or annoyance at being dependent, may help to put patients more at ease.

Nurse: I know that this may be hard for you, but remember that it is part of our work to help people who are ill. If there is anything that you would prefer to have done by someone else, let me know.

Offering some choices to the patient can help to restore a measure of dignity.

Talking about dying

Talking to people about dying or the fact that no more can be done to alter the course of illness is possibly the most challenging aspect of health care. Some doctors may find it hard to shift their treatment from curative to palliative care. Equally, some relatives and friends may show their reluctance to 'allow' the person to die by encouraging him to fight on to live. This may be stressful and upsetting for some patients, who, after an extended period of failing health, may welcome the relief from pain and suffering. Talking about dying and responding to people who seek hope and reassurance is challenging. Some patients are ambivalent about wanting to know the 'real' answers to their questions and ask them of people whom they do not expect to have the answers. Patients may ask questions of nurses that they do not put to doctors. The nurse might seem a more approachable member of the health care team because he spends far more time with the patient. An extract from a conversation illustrates the point:

Patient: When will I die?

Nurse: It is not possible to know that. How might it help you if we could tell you?

Patient: It wouldn't really, but I don't want to go on like this.

Nurse: What could we do or say to make you feel better or more comfortable?

Patient: Just keep me out of pain and make sure that I am not alone.

Nurse: We will do all we can to keep you comfortable. You will have to let us know when you are in pain. You say you don't want to be alone. Who would you most want to be with you?

Patient: My mother.

Nurse: Does she know this?

Patient: Not really. I haven't spoken to her in that way.

Nurse: Do you think you could talk to her more easily now?

Patient: I might today if I feel like it when she comes.

Nurse: If your mother isn't with you for any reason we will see that you are not alone.

Counsellors, especially nurses, find it easier to respond to patients' questions about their prognosis when the decision has been reached that only palliative care is to be provided.

Coming to terms with death

Health care providers and family members may assume that 'coming to terms with illness and death' is *necessary* and *desirable* for the patient's psychological well-being. This notion emanates from theories that view the denial of problems as being detrimental to psychological health. The way one person adjusts to or copes with what is happening to him may be very different from how another makes these adjustments.

A terminally ill patient may well connect the process of coming to terms with dying with an attempt to come to terms with how he has lived (see Chapter 6). Examples of some ideas that can be used in counselling if patients want to talk about death or dying are:

In whose life did the patient play a significant role?

Whose beliefs and ideas about living are most similar to his?

Who does he think will miss him most?

Does he have any regrets? What are these regrets?

What aspects of how he lived might make dying easier?

In our experience, many patients adjust to their deteriorating health in a way that differs from how they imagined they would behave. This may be due to their own inner resources and possibly the unexpected support from family and friends. As his health deteriorates, it is helpful to discuss the patient's needs with him and to provide opportunities to talk about the changes in his conditions and relationships over time. In the course of the conversation the counsellor may approach the subject as follows:

Counsellor:	John, tell me how you have managed this long period of illness as well as you have? What is it that helps you to keep going?
Patient:	I just live from hour to hour and day to day. I've decided that if I let myself think about the future it makes it hard for me to be calm about what is happening to me.
Counsellor:	So how do you manage to keep out thoughts about the future?
Patient:	I keep busy by seeing friends, and watching television a lot of the time.

Feelings of hope and hopelessness

During the terminal phase of illness, feelings of hopelessness stem from the certain knowledge that the 'end will inevitably come'. These feelings are sometimes accompanied by feelings of helplessness. There are two distinct aspects of hope in the terminal phase of HIV disease; physical and emotional hope.

Physical hope about the progress of the illness may be reflected in questions such as: 'Will it be slow or quick?' 'Will I be in pain?', and 'How uncomfortable will I be?' Close contacts and health carers may find this phase of palliative care very difficult if ideas and practices that accompany a 'good death' are not made clear by discussion with the patient. Doctors may feel under pressure to help the patient and others to maintain hope at all stages of illness. Some measure of hope *can* be maintained, but a careful choice of words is important if patients are not to be falsely reassured. One way of addressing the inevitability of death is to find out from patients what they know about their condition and how they want to be cared for. For example:

Counsellor:	What have the doctors told you about what's happening to you?
Patient:	I have a feeling they've given up hope.
Counsellor:	What makes you think that?
Patient:	They don't come to see me any more.
Counsellor:	Would you like them to come more often?
Patient:	I suppose so.
Counsellor:	Has anyone else given up hope?
Patient:	I'm in a daze now. I don't know what to think.
Counsellor:	Is there anything you hope for?
Patient:	Some quiet on the ward at night so I can sleep. More honesty from the doctors.
Counsellor:	How do you think you can influence the doctors to be more honest?
Patient:	Ask them more questions, I suppose. Actually, I hope they don't say to me 'it's the end'. It's OK feeling it, I just don't want to *hear* it.

The second aspect of hope relates to the patient's *emotional concerns*. Future questions may be used in conjunction with the patient's own genogram, if he is well enough, to address his hopes, for example, about being remembered after death. Helping patients to feel reassured that they may be remembered after death may in itself be a form of hope for them, and may ease the physical aspects of illness. A patient's hope that he will be remembered after death, and how he will be remembered, is very different from the hope that he may live longer, have a less painful death and not lose control. By encouraging a patient to talk about how he may be remembered, a counsellor may help a patient to feel hopeful in the face of imminent death. An excerpt from a conversation is used to illustrate the use of some future questions:

Counsellor: Was there anything special you wanted to talk about today?
Patient: It bothers me that I'm still frightened in some ways.
Counsellor: Can you try and say what is frightening you now?
Patient: Not having control now.
Counsellor: Would talking to people about how you would like to be remembered help you to feel you had some control?
Patient: Perhaps. I want to be remembered like I used to be, which was very much in control of my life.
Counsellor: By whom would you most want to be remembered like that?
Patient: My boyfriend, George, and also my parents. I hate them seeing me like this.
Counsellor: If you were to ask your partner which memory of you he might have in years to come what do you think he would say?
Patient: Maybe always making the decisions about where we should go on holiday.
Counsellor: Is this how you would like him to remember you?
Patient: Yes, because we had some really good times. He is never able to decide where to go.
Counsellor: Do you think he has learnt anything from you about making decisions?
Patient: I suppose he has. That you always have to take some risk in making decisions. Often these risks turn out to be worthwhile!

Saying 'goodbye'

There are rituals for ending relationships. Saying 'goodbye' to someone who is dying can be the most painful farewell. Relatives and friends may seek a counsellor's support and advice at this point. Brief but frequent visits to the patient, with short statements, may be all that is appropriate at this stage. However, if patients indicate that they have any concerns they should be helped to express them.

Counsellor: You say that your main concern is your worry that your father will 'go to pieces' when you die. Is there anything that will help you to not feel so worried?

Patient: No. I am ready to die and he won't let me go.

Counsellor: Have you been able to say this to him?

Patient: No. I couldn't.

Counsellor: Do the two of you usually have difficulty in saying what you want to each other?

Patient: Yes.

Counsellor: Do you think your father might 'let go' in his own time when he is ready? If he does it too soon, it may not be right for him.

Patient: Maybe I'll die before he's 'let go'.

Counsellor: Do you think that would be more difficult for your father or for you?

Patient: For him.

Counsellor: What would he have to do to show you he had 'let go'?

Patient: Not keep pushing food at me.

Counsellor: Do you think a father could *ever* let his child 'go'?

Patient: I suppose not. Maybe I should tell him I'm ready; that may help him a bit, which may help me.

Relatives can be reassured that just being there with the patient, sitting, holding a hand or reading, conveys closeness and a sense of relationship. In some instances, relatives and friends feel afraid and do not wish to be with the patient at the time of death. They may need 'permission' not to witness the death. The nurse in the following example does not put any pressure on the boyfriend of a dying patient to stay at his bedside.

Nurse: David is not very well tonight. What do you want us to do if his condition deteriorates further?

Partner: I would like to know, of course. Actually in my mind I have already said 'goodbye' to him. I don't know if I want to see him worse or dying.

Nurse: That is OK. It's been a really tiring day for you. Why don't you leave things with us for a while? We will give you a call at home if things change. You can decide then what you want to do.

CONCLUSION

The terminal phase of illness holds special challenges for the counsellor. There may be physical, practical, psychological and emotional concerns that patients may want to discuss or settle. As the patient becomes very ill, the counsellor may need to focus more attention on the close family and friends. Death ends a relationship in one sense, but at the same time, memories and ideas about the deceased may continue and affect those left behind. This paves the way for bereavement counselling, where required, and helps to promote emotional healing. In the next chapter we discuss bereavement counselling, which is inextricably linked to the theory discussed in this chapter.

SIXTEEN

Bereavement Counselling

I believe that the whole notion of 'healing' others (no less 'curing' them) is the most willful notion among helpful professionals. If it is to mean anything beyond symptom relief, healing must be a self-regenerative process.

Edwin Friedman

INTRODUCTION

It may be the painful feelings that come from loss and change following death that prompt people to seek professional counselling. While death is a part of every life-cycle, the untimely death of a child before his parents is a reversal of the natural order.

It is at the point of the patient's death that counselling for those left behind starts. The process of grieving may last for many months or years. For some who are bereaved a single counselling session may be sufficient to clarify their thoughts and feelings and to reassure them that they are coping as best they can under the circumstances. For others, several sessions, spaced over time and possibly with longer intervals between them, might be more appropriate. Sessions over a few years may be indicated at important dates, such as birthdays, anniversaries, or the anniversary of the death. There are some bereaved people who need to be seen more frequently.

As counsellors, we give the bereaved the opportunity to choose the intervals between counselling sessions. This is a useful way of gauging the bereaved person's perception of how he is coping and the level of anxiety he is experiencing, and we discuss this with him. It may be appropriate for counsellors to refer a bereaved person to a colleague who did not counsel during the terminal phase. Some bereaved people do not want to return to the place where the death occurred because of the associations it has for them. In some other circumstances the original counsellor may not be able to take on the specialist work that bereavement counselling entails.

WHY OFFER BEREAVEMENT COUNSELLING?

Counselling may be relevant at the stage of bereavement for a variety of reasons. Bereaved people can be helped to discuss and reflect on the changes brought about by loss. Information about the transmission of infection can be provided at this stage, as some bereaved people may lack knowledge about this or have unresolved fears for themselves or others. A counsellor can enable people to identify the effects of the loss and address these losses which is a way of looking towards the future. Although this process is distinct from that of 'coming to terms with the loss', it at least helps the bereaved to understand the loss in the context of day-to-day living.

Some people may never completely come to terms with a loss, particularly if it is the death of a child. The counsellor can help bereaved people to address the secrecy and social stigma associated with HIV infection, and to isolate these problems from the grief of bereavement. The bereaved person may feel socially isolated, and there is a danger that the counsellor can become his main social support as he may be the only other person who shares the secret about the causes of death and may have been there at the time of death.

The special circumstance of an HIV-infected survivor having to live with the same life-threatening condition as the deceased can be addressed through counselling, in order to introduce some ideas of hope and balance into the life of the bereaved. In addition, grieving may be more difficult when there have been multiple losses of friends through HIV disease. If losses come at frequent intervals, healing may be hampered by the lack of time, which is an essential part in the healing process.

TASKS IN COUNSELLING THE BEREAVED

A counselling task is to respond to grief reactions which may be masked. Sometimes the bereaved continue to live as if their relative or friend has not died, as they may find it too painful to think about the loss in case their feelings become overwhelming. Such reactions to loss and death, over a long period of time, can affect people's ability to manage their life on a day-to-day basis. If this apparent denial of reality is not addressed, it may become a problem that requires professional help. The bereaved's chances of becoming 'emotionally stuck' can be reduced by helping them to develop different ideas about what has happened in the past and new ideas about the future. The intense feelings which the survivors experience at the time of death may lead to later emotional or psychological problems.

HOW TO COUNSEL THE BEREAVED

Guidelines are set out to highlight ideas and themes which can be addressed in bereavement counselling. The counsellor's skill rests in his ability to weave these ideas into the conversation in a way that is appropriate for the individual, the nature of his problem and for the stage of bereavement that individual has reached.

The events leading up to the death

The circumstances of every death will affect people in different ways, and the counsellor should seek information about the facts of the death so as to help the survivors cope. Some of this information may already be known to the counsellor who has been involved with the patient and his contacts during the terminal phase of care. It may be therapeutic for the bereaved to talk about the events surrounding the death from a new perspective. The counsellor is able to provide an opportunity for the bereaved person to talk about painful feelings and secrets in an empathic environment. The counsellor can do this by exploring some of the following:

How long the deceased person was ill before dying.

Who else the deceased and the bereaved talked to about the illness.

From whom the deceased and bereaved got their support.

Whether it was a sudden death.

What provision was made for practical affairs before dying.

How the dying person prepared others, if at all, for his death.

What beliefs the deceased and bereaved had about living and dying.

Talking about the death

The way in which an individual died may leave memories that have an important effect on the bereaved. If, for example, the deceased choked to death, the bereaved may metaphorically remain 'choking with grief' (Andolfi *et al.*, 1983). If the person died peacefully, the memory might be of a 'good' death. In circumstances where the death took place surrounded by those the patient most loved, the view may be that he was not 'lonely'. Conversely, if the person died on his own in the night, it might be difficult for the bereaved to accept the reality of the death.

The counsellor may confirm that some of the bereaved's feelings of upset, grief or pain are expected and 'normal' and appropriate to that stage in the mourning process. In our experience, many people express great relief on hearing this.

Bereaved partner: I do still get upset. At times I don't know how I will manage from day to day.

Counsellor: I'd be surprised if you didn't feel that way. It is really quite normal at this stage.

Bereaved partner: That's true.

Counsellor: How long do you think this will go on? What do you think will have to happen to tell you that it will be time to start going out more often with your friends?

Rituals and events immediately after the death

The events that take place immediately after death may leave a lasting impression on the bereaved. The activities carried out can start or retard the mourning and healing process. Rituals can be followed to help the bereaved deal with overwhelming and incapacitating grief, and are traditionally a way of coping. A counsellor may help, for example, by suggesting to someone overwhelmed with grief that he sets aside time each day, in the morning and evening, to think about his relationship with the deceased and to imagine having a conversation with him. During the rest of the day he should not allow himself to think about the deceased person. In this way grieving is prescribed, in the hope that, when the person is not thinking about his grief, he may be enabled to have thoughts unrelated to the deceased (Selvini-Palazzoli *et al.*, 1977).

Rituals that surround death and the period after a death help people to confront and deal with the pain of the event. Such traditional activities provide a context in which mourning can take place, as well as assembling friends and relatives who provide social support. Religious ceremonies and customs have their place in coping with loss. In the Jewish religion, for example, people mourn actively and in varying degrees of intensity for a year. The period of bereavement is circumscribed and the bereaved person is expected to stop mourning and resume a normal life after this period. Some traditions prepare a feast which includes the favourite foods of the deceased person. Keeping a lock of hair or maintaining the deceased person's possessions are forms of memorials. A visit to the graveside or place of remembrance can also serve as a ritual. The 'Names Project', which started in the USA for those who died of AIDS, commemorates the life of the person in a patchwork quilt.

Bereavement counselling can, in its own right, take the place of a ritual for some people, as the conversations in counselling may keep alive memories of the deceased and provide a set time for expressing grief. Rituals may not be necessary or appropriate for everyone, since they have no meaning for some people. Counselling can help to uncover whether adherence to ritual holds meaning for a bereaved person, and therefore whether it can be helpful. Referring to the mourning activities as a healing process can in itself be therapeutic. The following questions will help clarify the rituals that were meaningful for the bereaved person:

Who took main responsibility for organizing the funeral?

Who made contact with family and friends?

Who was the most difficult person to tell?

What made it difficult to tell him?

Was there a religious ceremony? What did this mean to them?

Was anyone not told about the death, or not notified about the funeral? Who were they? What was the reason for not notifying them?

What beliefs were held about the deceased and 'after life'?

Who seemed most upset, and what were they upset about?

Who did the bereaved see most immediately after the death?

Who was most able to comfort the bereaved?

Was there any relief? What was related to this relief?

THEMES FOR THE SESSION

Some approaches for the counsellor include reference to previous experience of loss, present and past relationships, family of origin and family of choice, beliefs, thoughts about the past, present and future, the mourning process, and the use of genograms.

Coming for professional help

The point at which people come for professional help for bereavement may signal that they have become 'stuck'. It is important from a therapeutic point of view to note the point in the person's life-cycle at which he has become 'stuck', as it is helpful for the counsellor to understand whether there are other changes taking place that present as crises in the mourning process. For instance, if the bereaved is not able to look towards the future because he is constrained by the memories and pain of the past, he might now have to make a decision about whether to commit himself to a new relationship. For this reason, talking about the future may be as painful as talking about the past. Bereaved people may feel isolated because they are alone, or because others encourage them to 'look on the bright side'. Counselling may facilitate the expression of thoughts and fears that otherwise would not be spoken about. Where death has been unexpected or difficult to accept, talking about it may help to confirm this painful reality and make it more real for the bereaved.

Starting the session

The counsellor may discuss how best he can be of help to the bereaved. Recalling memories and thoughts about the deceased can sometimes help the bereaved to start talking about himself. To assess how he has been coping, the counsellor can enquire about how the bereaved person is spending his time. Thoughts about the future can be introduced by asking how he might have spent his time if he had not been grieving. Some examples of questions that can be used to initiate such discussion are:

How much of the time do you think about John?

You say that you think about John every evening just as you are about to go to sleep. Do these thoughts prevent you from going to sleep?

If you allowed yourself to forget his death for a while, what would you think about?

You say you'd feel disloyal if you didn't go to the cemetery. Where does this idea of disloyalty come from?

What memories of Frank do you most want to keep alive?

The following extract from a conversation with an HIV-infected bereaved partner illustrates some ways of helping him to talk about his fears for himself.

Partner:	I find Ivor's death frightening.
Counsellor:	What about it frightens you, Daniel?
Partner:	Well, as you know, I'm going to go the same way, and I just couldn't face all that suffering.
Counsellor:	As you know, Daniel, not everyone suffers in the same way, nor necessarily gets the same illnesses. Is there anything that you would do, or like to be done differently for yourself?
Partner:	I know that it might not be exactly the same. I have been coming regularly to the clinic, and, as you know, Ivor would not take any medicines that the doctors recommended. I have a slightly different view of that.
Counsellor:	At the moment you are well, Daniel. I can only say that we are here if there is anything you want to talk about, and if you have worries tell us so that we can see if any can be relieved.

An example of how the death of a father has affected the family, and how the counsellor can help the family to remember his beliefs and values is given below:

Counsellor:	We've spoken a lot about how this family has been different since your husband died. In what way is it the same?
Mother:	My son continues to help me whenever he can.
Counsellor:	How is this the same?
Mother:	I suppose he saw his father always helping me, and his own mother, especially when she was so frail.
Counsellor:	If your husband could see what was happening in your family today, what might his views be?
Mother:	He'd be pleased that the children were remembering some of the things that were important to him.

Previous experience of loss

If the bereaved person has had other experiences of loss it may influence how he deals with the loss in question. The idea of loss may be extended to encompass losses other than through death, such as loss through divorce, or the loss of the family through emigration. Helping the bereaved to make a connection with how they previously managed this loss may give them more confidence in their present ability to overcome the grief.

Counsellor:	Have you had personal losses before?
Bereaved:	Not the same as this. My father died suddenly four years ago.

Counsellor: How did you manage at that time?

Bereaved: I was very shocked as he was very fit. It took me a long time to believe it.

Counsellor: So was there anything from your father's death and how you coped that might help you now?

Bereaved: I suppose I know that over time the pain seems to lessen. I was more prepared for Sarah's death because I knew she had AIDS. Although I tried not to think it would end this way, I actually knew it would.

Where there have been multiple losses either in a family or of friends with HIV, 'shell shock' and emotional numbing may result. Helping the bereaved to express their feelings and concerns, as well as linking them with their previous experience of loss, can be a way of helping them to emerge from the shock.

Counsellor: What makes it so difficult for you to talk about John?

Partner: Just that he had to die.

Counsellor: If you were to let yourself talk about John, what might be the easier things to talk about and what might be the most difficult?

Partner: It is easier to talk about our relationship, which was really good. But it's also hard because there have been so many deaths and it might be my friend Jeremy next.

Counsellor: What have you learned from your experience of other friends that now might help you to deal with John's death?

Partner: That somehow it seems that people are not afraid when it comes to the end.

Counsellor: Then how can this help you with your own feelings?

Partner: Knowing that people I have known were not afraid at the end gives me some strength.

Present and past relationships

It is common for the bereaved to feel that it will be impossible for him to enjoy another enduring relationship. If he is not helped to address this belief or fear, he may lose confidence in his ability to enter into other relationships at some point in the future. Helping the bereaved person to look again at his relationship with the deceased sometimes rekindles the will to meet others. The following is a session with a bereaved partner:

Counsellor: Sarah, you tell me you feel quite lost without Clive. How do you see yourself carrying on without him?

Sarah: It is hard to think that I could ever make a close relationship again. I have a few friends. One in particular.

Counsellor: How does Clive's death affect your present relationships?

Sarah: I am frightened to get involved again in case I have to lose that person again.

Counsellor: What was learned from your relationship with Clive that might help you to decide to have a new relationship in the future?

Sarah: We were such good friends, even before we became lovers, and I know that is important.

Family of origin and family of choice

At times of death, a bereaved person may revive thoughts about his connections with the family of his partner who died. This in itself can be a source of pain if the relationship was not good (Walker, 1991). For example:

Counsellor: How did you, as Eric's boyfriend, get on with the family?
Partner: Hardly at all, because they didn't know about our relationship. They thought I was a good friend of Eric's.
Counsellor: Now that his mother has been told that you were more than a good friend, has that changed things in any way?
Partner: At first she was very friendly and I used to phone her once a week just like Eric did.
Counsellor: You said that at first it was better; what has happened since?
Partner: I don't know, but I guess she is mad that I got the flat.
Counsellor: How have you reacted to her being much less friendly?
Partner: I very seldom phone her.
Counsellor: So for whom is that more of a problem? You or her?
Partner: More her I think. She's very lonely.

Beliefs

Beliefs of the bereaved influence their perception of relationships and how people live from day to day. Beliefs about loyalty to family members, ideas about sex, marriage, and parent–child relationships may be re-evaluated when there is a death. The rituals surrounding death can serve to reveal, confirm or challenge beliefs. For instance, the idea that only the close family should be present at the funeral, and that gay partners do not have a right to their grief and sorrow can be brought into sharp focus. Counselling can help people to express the belief, its origins, and how it affects the bereaved. Some further examples of beliefs are:

No one will be able to grow and develop. Hidden behind a mother's grief may be the fear that she sees no future for the family.

A fear that '*too much upset*' will lead to a breakdown or mental illness, therefore it is better 'to keep the lid on'.

An idea that one has to be *loyal to the beliefs of others* such as parents and grandparents, by not showing emotion nor talking about feelings.

The following illustrates how to identify beliefs:

Counsellor: Where does the idea come from that you cannot show some relief after your sister's death?
Sister: It wouldn't seem right after all her suffering. My mother cried for six months after my father died. She was inconsolable.

Counsellor: What do you think that meant for all of you?
Sister: We were all too terrified to lighten things up. Mother would have thought that we were being disloyal. I would like to think that we needed to be like this to stop us all from cracking up.

Talking about the past, present and future (Chapter 3) links the bereaved's beliefs and ideas with death and loss. The counsellor has a special task in actively addressing with the bereaved aspects of the past which help them to look to the future. For example:

Counsellor: Which of your memories about Charles are the most important for you now?
Mother: Charles' wish for independence and his love of life.
Counsellor: What will that mean for you in the future?
Mother: I am not very independent and he always wanted me to do more things on my own. I might remind myself of his strengths and try and get out a bit more.

The mourning process

Adequate mourning is an essential part of the healing process. The counsellor can address this aspect with the bereaved. Positively encouraging mourning activities such as crying, wanting to be alone, thinking of the deceased, will allow the bereaved to grieve more freely and openly and accept the idea of death as a reality. It may also be useful to discuss mourning within certain time frames, thus giving some structure to what could otherwise seem to be an infinite process. Further, the counsellor could point out that, while mourning is an essential part of the healing process, excessive mourning could become a problem rather than part of the solution. The counsellor may want to see the bereaved from time to time to assess for himself how the mourning process is proceeding and to discuss its progression with the bereaved. It is equally important to recognize that not everyone has to go through this process, and not to impose on those who have suffered a death that this process is inevitable or necessary.

Genograms

The use of a genogram, that is, a drawing of a family tree which identifies relationships and patterns of relationships across and between generations, may be a powerful therapeutic intervention with the bereaved (Carter and McGoldrick, 1989). A genogram is a graphic representation of family history and relationships, as well as indicating closeness and distance between these relationships. Furthermore, it is a method of opening discussion about change, loss and patterns of support. In systemic counselling it can be an effective and compelling method of engaging people in a counselling session.

Genograms help to generate some interest in people's past and present, and can make them curious about their future. Constructing a genogram makes clearer and more immediate any discussion about loss, relationships and emotional attachments. Young children as well as adults can be readily engaged in this task. Genograms may be used to illustrate how beliefs, values and ideas have been passed down through generations. A method for doing this in clinical practice is described by McGoldrick and Gerson (1985).

A counsellor would start by asking the patient about those individuals who play an important part in his life. Using an established convention of mapping family composition and structure, the counsellor draws a family tree. Information that is relevant to the genogram is elicited by asking questions about relationships within the family.

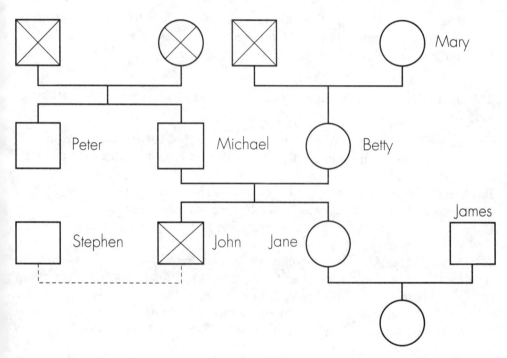

Figure 16.1 *Family genogram.*

Four generations of the family are shown on the genogram. John (28) died of AIDS. He had a six-year relationship with his boyfriend, Stephen, who was HIV-negative. The main themes explored with John's parents when they first came for bereavement counselling were:

(a) Their concern that the family name would not continue.
(b) The secret surrounding the sexual orientation of John's paternal uncle Peter.
(c) Support through the mother–daughter relationships (Betty and her mother Mary and her daughter Jane).
(d) The changing nature of Stephen's relationship to John's family after his death.

More complex themes emerged during the counselling as new connections were made between events and ideas.

Ending bereavement counselling

One aim of bereavement counselling is to help the bereaved reach a point where they are able more comfortably to look to and plan for the future. The ability to do this is an important indication that the period of mourning is drawing to a close. At this point, bereaved people may talk less about the deceased or they may start to think about new activities or relationships. The counsellor can assess the progress in bereavement counselling by identifying whether these changes have taken place, such as a return to previous routines or embarking on new activities. These may indicate that the end of bereavement counselling can be agreed upon.

Counsellor: What would tell you that your husband is beginning to see things differently since James' death?

Bereaved parent: When he starts to go to the pub again and can talk to his old mates.

The counsellor may explore and discuss the ending of bereavement counselling as follows:

Counsellor: We have spoken a lot about the things that have happened in your family since Sheila died. What effect do you think this has had on the family?

Brother: It has been difficult, but I think that it has brought us closer.

Counsellor: In what way do you think it has brought you closer?

Brother: We phone each other every week, and we get together at least once a month.

Counsellor: Has there been anything good about that?

Brother: I can't speak for everyone else, but I feel I have not been on my own in all this. Now I can talk to my mother about things that I have never been able to before. In fact, sometimes I think that I just repeat what I say here with you to the family. I was wondering if I really need to come so often.

CONCLUSION

The theories and approaches to bereavement counselling have a central part in HIV counselling generally as they draw on the experience of loss, which is relevant at all stages of HIV infection and illness. The death of a person from AIDS may give rise to new problems for those left behind, who may seek counselling.

The main tasks in bereavement counselling are to help the bereaved person to identify and address his principal concerns, to help him to mourn appropriately, and to enable him to look to the future. Counselling can help bereaved people to talk about events and painful feelings that might be difficult to discuss with relatives and friends. It is important to recognize that it might not be appropriate to offer ongoing bereavement counselling in certain settings, such as hospitals, because it may be detrimental to the process of recovery for the bereaved to return to the place where death occurred. Although aspects of bereavement counselling can be carried out by a range of health care providers, it is essentially a counselling task which demands specialized skills and, for this reason, should be provided only by those with the appropriate training and experience.

PART THREE

MEDICAL ASPECTS

SEVENTEEN

Medical Aspects of HIV Infection

Dr S.B. Squire, BSc, MRCP, Clinical Research Fellow and Honorary Senior Registrar

Dr M.A. Johnson, MD, MRCP, Consultant Physician in HIV/AIDS

Department of Thoracic Medicine and University Division of Communicable Diseases, Royal Free Hospital and School of Medicine, Pond Street, London NW3 2QG

INTRODUCTION

It is more than ten years since the acquired immunodeficiency syndrome (AIDS) was first recognized as a new clinical entity and it has been the subject of intense medical and scientific investigations. In these ten years physicians have moved from recognizing a particular constellation of opportunist infections and malignancies as AIDS to an understanding that this constellation is the end product of a progressive and relentless destruction of the human immune system caused by infection with human immunodeficiency viruses (HIV). The tenor of medical intervention has therefore moved from crisis management of illness as it arises to monitoring, early treatment and introduction of prophylactic regimes where possible.

VIROLOGY, IMMUNOLOGY AND LABORATORY DIAGNOSIS OF HIV INFECTION

Two genetically different human immunodeficiency viruses are now recognized as causative agents in AIDS: HIV-1 and HIV-2. HIV-1 is more prevalent worldwide and was identified before HIV-2. Consequently, most of our understanding of HIV infection is based on studies of HIV-1. Broadly speaking, however, the principal features of the viruses are the same: both are retroviruses whose prime target is the human CD4-lymphocyte and both contain their genetic information in the form of ribonucleic acid (RNA). These are important points for the understanding of the

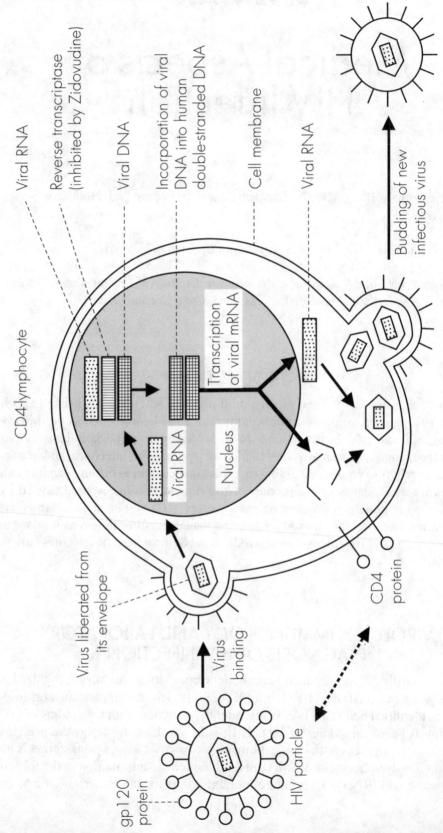

Figure 17.1 *HIV replication – schematic representation*

course of HIV infection. CD4-lymphocytes form a sub-population of the T-lymphocyte group that plays a crucial role in the majority of immune responses. Most of the opportunist infections and malignancies that arise in AIDS do so as a consequence of the progressive depletion of CD4-lymphocytes that is so clearly seen in HIV infection. The HIV virus particle binds to the CD4-lymphocyte through a specific interaction between one of its surface proteins (gp120) and the CD4 protein on the surface of the lymphocyte. This binding enables the virus to enter the lymphocyte. Through the action of a specific enzyme, reverse transcriptase, the virus then converts its RNA to deoxyribonucleic acid (DNA), which is then incorporated into the human DNA in the nucleus of the lymphocyte (Figure 17.1). The viral DNA is then in a position to be transcribed by human cellular enzymes, resulting in the production of viral proteins and, ultimately, the destruction of the lymphocyte and production of further viral particles. In a proportion of infected lymphocytes the viral DNA may not be transcribed immediately but is retained within the lymphocyte for transcription at a later date.

Immediately following initial infection of an individual with HIV, some of the protein products of viral replication may be detectable in blood samples, so-called HIV antigens. The predominant antigen is p24. At this stage it is uncommon for antibodies to HIV to be detectable, but these develop and become detectable in the vast majority of cases within three months of infection. This clearly has important implications for the diagnosis of HIV infection which rests, to a great extent, on the laboratory detection of HIV-specific antibodies in blood. Thus a patient may be infected with HIV and his or her body fluids will be potentially infectious before HIV antibodies are detectable in blood samples (see Figure 17.2). The duration of this 'window period' may be more than three months in a few exceptional cases (Haseltine, 1989; Ranki *et al.*, 1987) and this should be borne in mind when testing for HIV antibodies.

In practice, blood that is tested for HIV antibodies is first screened with an enzyme-linked immunoassay (ELISA). These ELISA tests are now extremely sensitive and specific (Squire *et al.*, 1991; Burke *et al.*, 1988). If this test proves reactive, confirmation of this is sought using other means of HIV-antibody detection such as Western blotting (Gallo *et al.*, 1986), immunoprecipitation (Squire *et al.*, 1991) or immunofluorescence (Gallo *et al.*, 1986) along with indirect evidence for HIV infection such as CD4 counting (Bofill *et al.*, 1992; Squire *et al.*, 1991). Newer methods may now make it possible to detect these antibodies in other body fluids, notably urine and saliva (Mortimer and Parry, 1992). Although separate and specific tests are needed to detect HIV-2, the principles of diagnosis are as described above for HIV-1. With the advent of nucleic acid amplification techniques it may eventually be possible to get away from detecting HIV antibodies and move towards detecting HIV nucleic acid sequences in HIV diagnosis (Loche and Mach, 1988).

The laboratory diagnosis of HIV infection presents particular problems in neonates and children. Infants born to HIV-seropositive mothers will initially have detectable HIV antibodies which they will have acquired passively from the

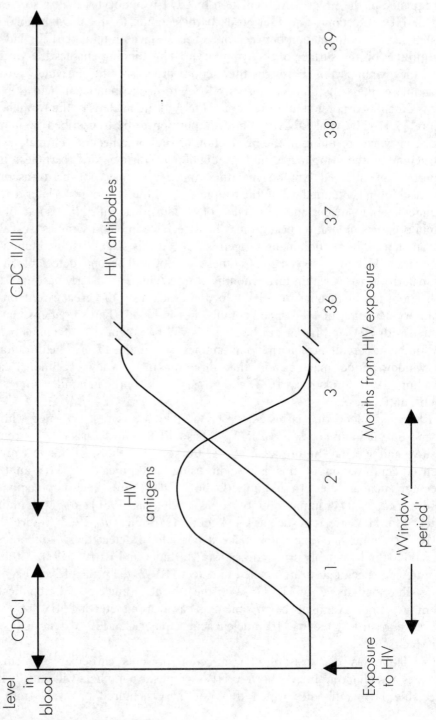

Figure 17.2 *Detection of HIV antigens and antibodies following infection.*

mother's circulation *in utero* (Hino *et al.*, 1987). These maternal antibodies may persist for up to 18 months and in that time period may not represent true HIV infection of the infant. True laboratory confirmation of HIV infection in a child therefore rests with the detection of HIV antibodies beyond 18 months of age or with the isolation of virus or viral protein products before this age (Hino *et al.*, 1987). It may eventually be possible to use sensitive nucleic acid amplification techniques to detect HIV DNA or RNA sequences in the blood of foetuses (obtained by cordocentesis *in utero*) or neonates. However, this is not yet technically possible (Laure *et al.*, 1988).

EPIDEMIOLOGY AND TRANSMISSION OF HIV INFECTION

HIV virus particles have been found in most body fluids (see Table 1) but epidemiological studies have established that the only important routes of transmission are via penetrative sexual contact (vaginal or anal intercourse), direct inoculation of blood (or untreated blood products) from HIV-infected individuals, and from mother to child *in utero* or perinatally (see Tables 2 and 3). There is no proof for transmission by social contact or biting insects such as mosquitoes. HIV is transmitted by both active and passive sexual intercourse but the risk is greater for the receptive or passive partner (male or female). HIV infection was therefore first recognized in individuals with many sexual partners (especially prostitutes and homosexual or bisexual men). There is evidence that transmission is more likely where there is a greater chance of direct contact with the blood circulation, as may occur when sexual intercourse is associated with trauma and bleeding or genital ulceration (O'Farrell, 1989). Regular use of condoms reduces this contact and therefore reduces the risks of transmission but does not provide 100 per cent protection. The transmission of HIV by inoculation of blood is usually seen in intravenous drug users who share injecting equipment but has also been demonstrated where contaminated needles or scalpels have been used in the health care setting (vaccination/injections/surgery) and in accidental needle-stick injuries (Marcus, 1988). Blood transfusion-related transmission is rarely seen in countries where donated blood is screened for HIV but may still occur in isolated cases because of the window period for the detection of HIV antibodies described above. Heat treatment of factor VIII and IX concentrates for haemophiliacs has halted the appearance of concentrate-related HIV infection in these patients.

Several patterns of predominant transmission have been recognized worldwide. In the developed world (Western Europe and North America) the greatest number of HIV-infected individuals has been identified among homosexual/bisexual men, intravenous drug users, and haemophiliacs. Increasingly, however, cases are recognized in the heterosexual population and recent data on the HIV seroprevalence in newborn infants point towards an increase of HIV infection in the general population. The main virus in this geographical area is HIV-1. In the developing world, the greatest number of cases has been seen in the heterosexual

Table 1 Body fluids from which HIV has been isolated

Blood
Semen
Cervical secretions
Saliva
Tears
Urine
Cerebrospinal fluid
Bronchoalveolar lavage fluid

Table 2 Proven routes for transmission of HIV

1. **Penetrative sexual intercourse**
   anal/vaginal
   increased transmission in presence of genital ulceration
   increased risk if associated with trauma/bleeding

2. **Direct inoculation of infected blood/blood products**
   Factor VIII in haemophiliacs
   infected blood in blood transfusions
   infected blood via sharp instruments/needles – e.g. intravenous drug users and health care workers

3. **Mother to child**
   in utero
   during delivery
   breast-feeding

Table 3 Routes for which there is no proof for HIV transmission

Social contact (hand-shaking, kissing on cheek)
Sharing cutlery
Sharing toilet facilities
Via biting insects (e.g. mosquitoes)

population and, consequently, in children. The situation is particulary grave in Africa, where one in forty adults are now infected with HIV (Sixth International Conference on AIDS in Africa, Dakar, 1991 (Potts, 1992)). Again, HIV-1 is the main virus identified, but an epidemic of immunodeficiency consequent on HIV-2 infection centred on West Africa has been identified and cases of HIV-2 infection have now been reported in many other parts of Africa and the rest of the world.

Epidemiological studies have established that between 13 per cent and 39 per cent of babies born to HIV-infected mothers will be truly HIV-infected (European Collaborative Study, 1991). These children will have acquired the virus either *in utero* (Courgnaud *et al.*, 1991) or from maternal body fluids during delivery (Ehrnst *et al.*, 1991). The relative importance of these two modes of transmission has not yet been defined. At present there is no evidence that elective delivery by caesarean section of mothers known to be HIV-infected will reduce the risk of transmission.

HIV-1 may also be transmitted by breast-feeding. Breast-feeding is the main mode of transmission of another human retrovirus, HTLV-1 (Hino *et al.*, 1987). At present, therefore, where adequate facilities are available for the feeding of artificial milk, this is advised for infants of HIV-infected mothers. However, it must be emphasized that in the countries where most HIV-infected mothers are identified, particularly in developing parts of Africa, the risks of feeding artificial milk far outweigh the risks of HIV infection by breast milk.

NATURAL HISTORY AND CLASSIFICATION OF HIV INFECTION

Classification of HIV infection in adults

As clinical patterns of disease were recognized in adults to be indicative of HIV infection, so clinical classifications of disease were developed to guide research, clinical trials and patient management. The Centers for Disease Control (CDC) in Atlanta, Georgia devised a system for defining AIDS cases (Table 4) (CDC, 1987a). This has been modified in various ways to meet geographical needs (Table 5) (De Cock *et al.*, 1992). The term AIDS-related complex (ARC) was coined to describe a series of clinical manifestations that indicated HIV infection but did not constitute full-blown AIDS. As serological tests for HIV antibodies became available a syndrome comprising various combinations of fever, rashes, diarrhoea, and neurological manifestations was recognized as being associated with acute HIV infection and became known as the HIV seroconversion syndrome. The CDC then provided a widely used system of classification (CDC, 1986) which divided HIV infection into four stages (see Table 6). With the recognition that certain laboratory indicators of immune function – notably blood CD4-lymphocyte counts – carried prognostic significance, these were incorporated into classification systems such as the Walter Reed system (Redfield *et al.*, 1986). Now, as physicians increasingly view HIV infection as a chronic viral disease with early and late stages and no truly asymptomatic phase, rather than a set of clinical syndromes arising suddenly as a result of activation of a latent viral infection, there have been calls to review the use of the clinical systems and incorporate laboratory prognostic markers in order to classify HIV infection as mild, moderate or severe (Paul Volberding, Sixth International AIDS Conference, Florence, 1991).

Prognostic markers

The impetus for this use of prognostic markers has arisen out of cohort studies of haemophiliacs (Phillips *et al.*, 1991), homosexual men (Phair *et al.*, 1990) and intravenous drug users (Moss and Bacchetti, 1989) which have clearly established that the average time of HIV infection from seroconversion to the development of

Table 4   Summary of CDC case definitions for AIDS in adults (CDC, 1987a)
(compare with Table 6)

For epidemiological surveillance an adult (> 13 years) is considered to have AIDS if one or more of the following conditions are diagnosed:

A   Constitutional disease
HIV wasting syndrome
B   Neurological disease
HIV encephalopathy ('AIDS dementia')
C   Symptomatic or invasive disease due to secondary infectious disease
  C-1   **Opportunist infectious disease**
    Pneumocystis carinii pneumonia
    chronic cryptosporidiosis
    toxoplasmosis
    extra-intestinal strongyloidiasis
    isosporiasis
    oesophageal, bronchial or pulmonary candidiasis
    cryptococcosis
    histoplasmosis
    mycobacterial infection with *M. avium intracellulare* or *M. kansasii*
    cytomegalovirus infection
    chronic mucocutaneous herpes simplex infection
    progressive multifocal leukoencephalopathy
  C-2   **Other infectious diseases**
    recurrent *Salmonella* bacteria
    mycobacterial infection with *M. tuberculosis* (involving at least one site outside the lungs)
D.   Secondary cancers
Kaposi's sarcoma
Non-Hodgkins lymphoma (small non-cleaved lymphoma or immunoblastic sarcoma)
primary lymphoma of the brain

immune-deficiency syndromes is ten years. Although it is not yet proven beyond doubt that all HIV-infected patients will develop AIDS in the absence of medical intervention, the indicators are that this will be the case (Moss and Bacchetti, 1989). The most widely recognized laboratory indicator of HIV progression is now the blood absolute CD4-lymphocyte count (Phillips *et al.*, 1991; Bofill *et al.*, 1992), but there are limitations for its use in children who have higher overall lymphocyte counts than adults (Bofill *et al.*, 1992) and in other situations where overall lymphocyte counts are changed, for instance in individuals of African origin, or in

Table 5   Suggested case definitions for AIDS in Africa
(De Cock *et al.*, 1992)

For epidemiological surveillance an adult (> 13 years) is considered to have AIDS if the CDC surveillance case definition for AIDS is fulfilled
  or
a test for HIV infection gives positive results
  and
one or more of the following are present:

> > 10 per cent body weight loss or cachexia, with diarrhoea or fever, or both, intermittent or constant, for at least one month, not known to be due to a condition unrelated to HIV infection

> Tuberculosis with the features given above, or tuberculosis that is disseminated (involving at least two different organs) or miliary, or extrapulmonary tuberculosis

> Kaposi's sarcoma

> Neurological impairment sufficient to prevent independent daily activities, not known to be due to a condition unrelated to HIV infection (e.g. trauma)

patients who have undergone splenectomy or who are receiving chemotherapy. Nonetheless, it is increasingly recognized that patients with CD4-lymphocyte counts less than $0.2 \times 10^9/l$ are at risk for development of opportunist infections (Crowe *et al.*, 1990; Phair *et al.*, 1990). It is often, therefore, helpful to view the progression of HIV infection as mirrored by the peripheral blood CD4-lymphocyte count, as indicated in Figure 17.3. An important feature to bear in mind in this sort of strategy is that CD4-lymphocyte counts will vary considerably within one individual according to such factors as time of day and concurrent illness or stress. Another limitation of CD4-lymphocyte counts is that, although they may help in guiding prognosis and medical intervention for asymptomatic patients, once opportunist infections develop and the CD4 counts fall below $0.2 \times 10^9/l$ their relevance is less clear. Nonetheless, a category of patients at particular risk with CD4 counts $< 0.05 \times 10^9/l$ is increasingly discussed.

Other laboratory markers are also in widespread use. Blood beta-2-microglobulin (B2M) levels are raised in all chronic viral infections and levels rise with the progression of HIV infections. B2M levels were shown to be more useful in predicting beneficial responses to Zidovudine therapy than CD4 counts in clinical trials (Jacobson *et al.*, 1991a). The presence of HIV antigens, and particularly p24 antigen, has been associated with worse prognosis. This marker has, however, the disadvantage that it does not become positive in all cases of AIDS and levels of antigenaemia may therefore only be of prognostic significance for the small subgroup of patients who have detectable levels. At this stage, other markers of disease progression such as neutralizing anti-gp120 antibodies, lymphocyte performance assays, highly specific anti-p24 antibodies, and neopterin levels are in use in

Table 6   Summary of CDC classification of HIV infection (CDC, 1986)
(Compare with Table 4)

Group I   Acute infection ('seroconversion')
Group II Asymptomatic infection
Group III Persistent generalized lymphadenopathy
Group IV Other disease

      A. Constitutional disease
      One or more of: fever > 1 month
                          involuntary weight loss > 10 per cent of baseline
                          diarrhoea > 1 month
      (in absence of causes other than HIV)

      B. Neurological disease
      One or more of: dementia
                          myelopathy
                          peripheral neuropathy
      (in absence of causes other than HIV)

      C. Secondary infectious disease
         C-1 **Opportunist**
            As for AIDS definition; see Table 4
         C-2 **Other**
            oral hairy leukoplakia
            multidermatomal herpes zoster
            recurrent *Salmonella* bacteraemia
            nocardiasis
            tuberculosis
            oral candidiasis

D. Secondary cancers
As for AIDS definition; see Table 4

E. Other conditions
e.g. neoplasms other than those in D, or recurrent infections other than those in C

---

individual centres and have not yet received the widespread evaluation given CD4-lymphocyte counting, B2M and HIV antigens.

As already mentioned, the laboratory diagnosis of HIV infection in children presents particular difficulties. Similarly, the effect of HIV infection on the developing immune system appears to give rise to a few more clinical syndromes in children than those seen in adults. This is particularly exemplified by the development of lymphoid interstitial pneumonitis (LIP) in children, which is a rare development in adults. The paediatric case definition for AIDS therefore differs from that of adults and includes LIP and recurrent bacterial infection (CDC, 1987b). The same laboratory markers of HIV progression have been employed in children but have not been as extensively evaluated. As described above, overall

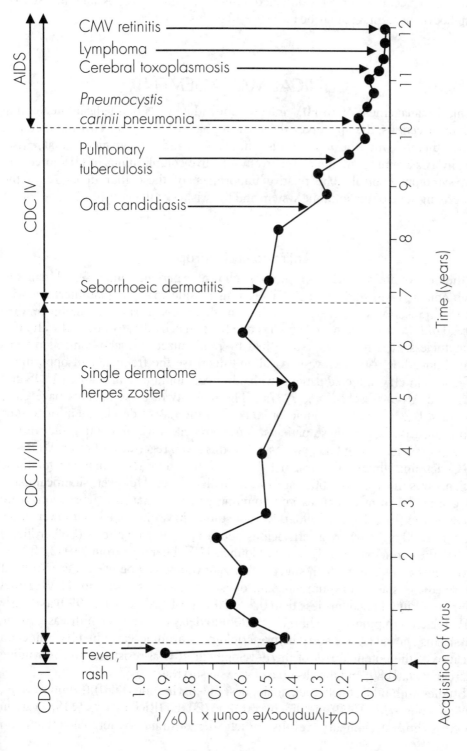

Figure 17.3 *Representative decline in CD4 count with progression of HIV infection.*

lymphocyte counts and, consequently, CD4-lymphocyte counts, are higher in infants than in adults and fall naturally with age (Bofill *et al.*, 1992). This must be taken into account for HIV-infected children, and it is possible that CD4-lymphocyte percentages may be more useful in this instance.

CLINICAL MANAGEMENT

Clinical management of an HIV-infected individual rests on medical intervention in four directions; therapy directed specifically against HIV (antiretroviral therapy), acute therapy for the opportunist infections and malignancies that arise, prophylaxis against common or recurrent infective complications of HIV infection, and symptom control. The relative importance of these four depends on the underlying state of the immune system and the wishes of the individual.

Antiretroviral therapy

In the field of antiretoviral therapy, most clinical experience and research data has been obtained with Zidovudine. This is a nucleoside analogue that interferes with reverse transcriptase activity. By definition, therefore, it can only inhibit onward spread of HIV from cell to cell and has no effect on cells already infected with HIV. Nonetheless, it is now well established by randomized, placebo-controlled trials that Zidovudine will improve survival and decrease the frequency of opportunist infections in HIV-infected patients with advanced immunocompromise (AIDS and advanced ARC) (Fischl *et al.*, 1987a). The majority of these patients have CD4 counts $< 0.2 \times 10^9$/l and, in accordance with the risk of development of serious opportunist disease in these patients, most physicians will now offer Zidovudine therapy to patients with CD4 counts below this level, regardless of prior AIDS- or ARC-defining illness. The original dose of Zidovudine recommended for these patients was in excess of 1000 mg/day in divided doses. However, significant side effects, in the form of nausea and vomiting and bone marrow depression, were encountered (Fischl *et al.*, 1990a). Recent studies have suggested that lower doses (400 mg–500 mg/day) are as efficacious but carry fewer side effects (Volberding *et al.*, 1990; Nordic Medical Research Council HIV Therapy Group, 1992). There have now been studies which suggest that Zidovudine can be used successfully at intermediate stages of immunocompromise in patients with no HIV-related symptoms but CD4 counts less than 0.5×10^9/l (Volberding *et al.*, 1990) and early HIV-related symptoms (Fischl *et al.*, 1990b) to delay progression of disease. Some physicians, however, are wary of prescribing Zidovudine early in HIV infection because of the potential risk of the development of viral resistance to Zidovudine (Larder *et al.*, 1989) and the absence of data on survival.

Studies with other nucleoside analogues, dideoxyinosine (DDI) (Lambert *et al.*, 1990; Cooley *et al.*, 1990) and dideoxycytidine (DDC) (Richman *et al.*, 1987) are in progress and preliminary results which demonstrate favourable effects on laboratory markers such as CD4 count are available. At this stage, however, there is no firm data in support of effects on survival or disease progression for these drugs. The principal side effects of these drugs (pancreatitis for DDI and peripheral neuropathy for DDI and DDC) have now been identified and dose ranges can be recommended. Trials using combinations of nucleoside analogues are planned, and it is hoped that these may lead to ways of averting viral resistance and reducing side effects.

Apart from interference with the reverse-transcriptase-dependent stage of HIV infection, other strategies for targeting HIV infection are under consideration: interfering with gp120-CD4 binding with soluble recombinant CD4 molecules, TIBO compounds, and various forms of immunotherapy. In this last category, the aim is to present HIV-specific antigens (proteins) to the immune system of HIV-infected individuals in such a way as to trigger an immune response that will lead to control of virus replication. At this stage, however, none of these has been of proven efficacy in the clinical situation.

Opportunist infections

In the developed world, *Pneumocystis carinii* pneumonia (PCP) is the predominant AIDS-defining illness and a major cause of morbidity and mortality in HIV-infected patients (Jacobson *et al.*, 1991b; Phair *et al.*, 1990). Prior to the AIDS epidemic some experience with treating this condition with high-dose systemic cotrimoxazole and pentamidine had already been gained in patients immuno-compromised by malignancy, chemotherapy or malnutrition. These drugs remain the mainstay of treatment of PCP in AIDS. Although newer drugs are under investigation (Falloon *et al.*, 1991), the major advances in this field since the advent of AIDS have been made in the diagnosis, general management and prophylaxis of the condition.

PCP usually presents with a history of a dry, non-productive cough associated, variably, with shortness of breath and fever. Unfortunately, conventional tests used for respiratory diagnosis in such patients (e.g. chest X-rays and pulmonary function tests) may only give an indication of the extent of pulmonary disease without giving information on the specific cause of the symptoms, be it an infectious agent or a structural problem such as endobronchial Kaposi's sarcoma. In many cases, therefore, a procedure is required to obtain samples of lung tissue for examination in the laboratory. The definitive procedure remains fibreoptic bronchoscopy with bronchoalveolar lavage and/or transbronchial biopsy (Metersky and Catanzaro, 1991). Some centres have, however, developed slightly less invasive techniques such as sputum induction by inhalation of an irritant aerosol (Leigh *et al.*, 1990). Depending on individual circumstances, physicians may use more or less invasive techniques from the outset or hold them in reserve for cases where empiric anti-pneumocystis therapy (e.g. with cotrimoxazole) fails.

Early in the epidemic it became clear that HIV-infected patients recovering from a first episode of PCP faced an increased risk of recurrence of the condition within six months. This risk has now been significantly reduced by the introduction of prophylactic regimes such as low-dose oral cotrimoxazole (Ruskin and LaRiviere, 1991) and nebulized pentamidine (Leoung *et al.*, 1990). On the basis of the increased risk of opportunist infection in patients with CD4 counts less than $0.2 \times 10^9/l$, and one placebo-controlled study showing that daily oral cotrimoxazole prevented the onset of PCP in patients with Kaposi's sarcoma (Fischl *et al.*, 1987b), it is now recommended that all HIV-infected patients receive some sort of prophylaxis against PCP once CD4 counts fall below this level, regardless of prior experience of PCP (CDC, 1989). Preliminary data from a comparative trial (AIDS Clinical Trials Group 021) suggest that low-dose oral cotrimoxazole has greater efficacy as secondary prophylaxis against PCP. Nebulized pentamidine seems to be associated with more failures of prophylaxis and costs more to deliver. In contrast, systemic cotrimoxazole is cheap, effective, and may provide prophylaxis against other infective complications such as toxoplasmosis. However, it may be associated with unacceptable systemic side effects in some patients. Most physicians agree that some sort of prophylaxis against PCP is important for patients with advanced immunocompromise and would now advise low-dose cotrimoxazole as first-line prophylaxis.

The second most common infectious agent identified in the lungs of severely immunocompromised HIV-infected patients is cytomegalovirus (CMV). However, it seems that this agent only contributes to significant lung dysfunction in a few special cases (Millar *et al.*, 1990; Squire *et al.*, 1992).

More significant worldwide is the problem of tuberculosis in HIV-infected patients. It is now well recognized that HIV infection is associated with an increased incidence of symptomatic infection with *Mycobacterium tuberculosis* (MTB). The majority of HIV-infected patients presenting with MTB have respiratory symptoms but some of the features of the disease differ when compared to classical pulmonary MTB in immunocompetent patients. For example, disease of the pleura is more common and more cases of MTB affecting organs other than the lung are seen (Harries, 1990). Presentations with MTB-associated disease tend to occur in patients with relatively preserved CD4-lymphocyte counts (in the range 0.2–$0.4 \times 10^9/l$ when compared with presentations with PCP. MTB-associated disease is not AIDS-defining unless there is evidence of systemic spread (see Table 4). It tends to respond well to conventional quadruple chemotherapy. The other tuberculous disease seen commonly in AIDS patients is that associated with *Mycobacterium avium intracellulare* (MAI). This, and other 'atypical' mycobacteria, can cause disease in any organ and tends to be a late manifestation in AIDS patients with very advanced immunocompromise. Response to conventional chemotherapy is variable but newer drugs are being used with some success.

With any severe respiratory disease in HIV-infected patients the question of life support with mechanical ventilation in an intensive care setting may arise. Although reviews of patient outcome in patients ventilated for PCP early in the epidemic were universally depressing (short-term mortality rates in excess of 50 per cent and no patients surviving more than one year), more recent results (Friedman *et al.*, 1991) and case reports are encouraging. This improvement is probably attributable to several features, including improvements in general management and disease recognition as well as introduction of steroid chemotherapy for severe cases of PCP (Bozette *et al.*, 1990; Gagnon *et al.*, 1990). Although individual decisions about life support will depend on many factors, including patients' wishes, most physicians will now recommend ventilation to patients with the first clinical manifestations of severe immunocompromise (such as a first episode of PCP). With the availability of less invasive forms of ventilatory support such as nasal intermittent positive pressure ventilation (Elliot *et al.*, 1990) it may be possible to avoid full ventilation in a number of cases.

Although PCP is the commonest AIDS-defining presentation in the developed world, most cases of AIDS in the developing world present with a history of relentless diarrhoea and weight loss. This presentation is also common in Europe and North America. In a number of cases it appears that HIV itself causes the diarrhoea. It is, however, important to obtain appropriate gut samples to identify causative agents that may respond to therapeutic regimes, as indicated in Table 7. In the simplest cases this will involve examination of stool samples for parasites and culture for viruses and bacteria, including mycobacteria. In other cases direct visualization and/or biopsy of the gut mucosa by procedures such as colonoscopy and gastroscopy may be required. Multiple samples may be needed to provide sufficient material for microbial culture as well as histological examination.

Table 7 Causative agents associated with diarrhoea in AIDS patients

AGENT	TREATMENT
cytomegalovirus	ganciclovir
cryptosporidium	spiramycin
M. avium intracellulare	quadruple chemotherapy as for *M. tuberculosis* (variable results)
Giardia lamblia	metronidazole
Entamoeba histolytica	metronidazole
Non-typhi *Salmonella*	cotrimoxazole
Campylobacter jejuni	erythromycin
Shigella	ampicillin
Isospora	cotrimoxazole
microsporidium	none

Although common pathogens such as *Campylobacter* and *Salmonella* causing diarrhoeal syndromes in AIDS may respond easily to conventional therapy, relapses or recurrences are common. This is also true of the opportunist infectious agents such as cytomegalovirus, cryptosporidium, and microsporidium. Treatment of these conditions tends to be more difficult.

Cryptosporidium and cytomegalovirus may also be associated with disorders of the biliary tree in the absence of diarrhoeal symptoms. Various infective agents may involve the liver and include the hepatitis viruses, cryptococcus and MAI. Liver biopsy may be needed for diagnosis.

Disorders of the mouth are common in HIV infection (Feigal *et al.*, 1991). Recurrent oral candidiasis (thrush) usually responds readily to local antifungal solutions as well as systemic therapies such as fluconazole or ketoconazole. Recurrent oral ulceration due to herpes simplex infection is also common and often requires systemic therapy with oral acyclovir. Gum infections and tooth decay may require specialist dental attention. A particular condition thought to be secondary to Epstein-Barr virus replication and known as oral hairy leucoplakia is commonly seen on the lateral borders of the tongue as white, corrugated plaques. Although pathognomonic of HIV infection, this condition is rarely symptomatic or invasive and carries little prognostic significance.

HIV-infected patients who present with loss of appetite and/or difficulty with swallowing require careful assessment as these symptoms may indicate the presence of oesophageal disorders. The commonest causes of these symptoms in AIDS patients are candida and cytomegalovirus oesophagitis. Upper gastro-intestinal endoscopy with biopsy is often required for adequate diagnosis especially as both candida and CMV oesophagitis are AIDS-defining. Both respond well to systemic therapy but may recur.

Neurological disease is one of the most feared consequences of HIV infection, and the threat of blindness from cytomegalovirus retinitis is a particular aspect of neurological disease in patients that requires much attention. This tends to be a late manifestation of HIV infection. Presenting symptoms include blurred vision and the reporting of floaters across the field of vision. Treatment is possible with either ganciclovir (Minor, 1991) or foscarnet (Palestine *et al.*, 1991). Unfortunately both these drugs have significant toxicities and require intravenous administration and long-term maintenance regimes which may require the placement of semi-permanent in-dwelling venous catheters. These may prove a troublesome source of bacterial infections.

Other opportunist infections of the central nervous system are a particular problem in HIV infection. The commonest presenting symptoms are persistent headache, fever and/or localizing neurological signs such as hemiparesis or loss of speech. In these instances computerized tomography (CT) or magnetic resonance imaging (brain-scanning) is needed to identify space-occupying lesions causing raised intracranial pressure before lumbar puncture is performed to examine cerebrospinal fluid for meningeal infections. Cryptococcal meningitis may present insidiously without the classic signs of meningeal irritation (neck stiffness and photophobia) but may respond well to therapy with amphotericin and flucytosine. It usually requires long-term suppressive therapy with fluconazole.

Toxoplasma gondii is the commonest infective cause of a space-occupying cerebral lesion in AIDS and, although the appearance on CT scanning may not be typical, a trial of anti-toxoplasma therapy (typically sulphadiazine and pyrimeth-amine) is usually indicated before more definitive diagnostic procedures such as brain biopsy (Holliman *et al.*, 1991) are carried out. Toxoplasmosis responds well to treatment; however, it frequently recurs and patients should receive life-long secondary prophylaxis. Progressive multifocal leukoencephalopathy (PML) caused by JC virus may take on similar appearances on CT scans to *Toxoplasma gondii* and may present similarly. Although the prognosis associated with PML is poor and there is no treatment of proven efficacy, there have been case reports of responses with cytarabine (Nicoli *et al.*, 1992).

In addition to the opportunist infections affecting the nervous system, HIV can itself cause damage to nerve tissue (Simpson and Wolfe, 1991). A syndrome of progressive memory and cognitive dysfunction (AIDS dementia) is well recognized and is probably caused by HIV replication in brain tissue. Zidovudine use in AIDS appears to have reduced the frequency of this condition (Fischl *et al.*, 1990b) but there are concerns that recent calls for reduction in Zidovudine dosage will lead to lower and less effective Zidovudine levels across the blood–brain barrier. HIV infection may also cause progressive loss of sensation and movement in limb extremities (peripheral neuropathy) or more localized nerve disorders (mono-neuritis multiplex, myelopathy). These tend not to respond to Zidovudine, and clinical management is directed at excluding more readily treatable causes such as vitamin deficiency, drug toxicity and, perhaps, CMV infection.

Malignancies in HIV

The central nervous system is also a common site for development of lymphomas in AIDS. B-cell non-Hodgkins lymphomas (BcNHL) are AIDS-defining in HIV-infected patients and are usually managed according to experience of lymphomas in the immunocompetent population. Prognosis is variable and generally seems to depend on the underlying state of immunocompromise at presentation. Other lymphomas, including T-cell and Hodgkins types, are increasingly recognized in HIV-infected patients but are not, as yet, AIDS-defining.

The classic AIDS-associated malignancy is Kaposi's sarcoma (KS). This is a disfiguring vascular tumour that seems to arise in a multicentric fashion more commonly than as a single lesion with local (or distant) metastases. In the developed world it presents in men who have acquired HIV by homosexual contact. It is rare in those infected by intravenous drug use, blood products or heterosexual contact. In the developing world, especially Africa, it is common in both sexes. These observations have led to speculation that it is caused by an unidentified sexually transmissible agent (Beral *et al.*, 1990). When KS presents as localized cutaneous lesions, local radiotherapy or intralesional injection of cytotoxic agents or interferon-alpha have been used to good effect. However, when the lesions are proliferating and/or systemic and detected in the lungs, gut or other viscera, the prognosis is poor and systemic chemotherapy is indicated. For patients who present with KS and reasonably preserved CD4-lymphocyte counts, response to daily subcutaneous or intramuscular injections of interferon-alpha is possible. This has the advantage of less bone-marrow toxicity than the standard chemothera-peutic regimes needed for patients with lower CD4-lymphocyte counts. As Zidovudine is indicated for patients with KS, this may be an important issue in deciding between the different regimes.

A number of malignancies that have been associated with transmissible agents and immunocompromise are also seen in HIV-infected patients. The frequency of cervical intra-epithelial neoplasia is increased in HIV-infected women and may be associated with papilloma virus infection. Conventional ablative techniques are employed but the true natural history of this condition in HIV is not known. A parallel condition which is occasionally encountered in homosexual, HIV-positive men is squamous cell carcinoma of the anal canal.

Terminal care

At some point in the medical management of HIV infection the emphasis shifts from active, and sometimes invasive, diagnosis and treatment to symptom control. The way in which this takes place depends very much on a patient's wishes and circumstances. It may be a difficult transition to make, not only as a state of mind for the patient, but for the physician as well. In many cases community care teams, including general practitioners, district nurses, hospice practitioners, family members, partners and friends, become especially important. If key members of these groups have not been involved in patient care at earlier stages in HIV infection the necessary relationships and understanding required for effective symptom control cannot develop. There is an important barrier here that must be overcome by both physicians and patients. In the earlier stages of HIV infection when patients have no symptoms, they see little need for contact with their general practitioner and little need for dissemination of information about their infection. While active diagnosis and treatment are being pursued, patients naturally turn to their investigating physicians, who are usually hospital-based. They may have continuing concerns about confidentiality and may ask hospital physicians to keep medical details from their general practitioners. Hospital physicians may collude with these attitudes. However, greater efforts need to be made to involve general practitioners and local community services at an early stage. The appointment of liaison staff, such as community nurse specialists, is facilitating this transition. At a practical level, control of pain, nausea and agitation may often need delivery of drugs by syringe drivers and requires trained supervision.

Clinical trials and prospects for the 1990s

In general, medical management in HIV infection is guided by an assessment of the underlying state of immunocompromise. This assessment is usually based on a combination of clinical history and examination and laboratory prognostic markers such as CD4-lymphocyte count. The relative emphasis given to these factors will depend on available expertise and experience. When an assessment indicates severe immunocompromise the emphasis of medical advice is on intervention with agents whose effects are already well documented. There is clearly also an obligation on medical staff to consider newer treatments and to discuss with their patients enrolment in clinical trials of these treatments. In the 1990s this will become increasingly important for patients with relatively preserved immune function. Most of the progress in clinical management of HIV in the last decade has been made in patients with advanced immunocompromise and symptoms.

Unfortunately, the urgency of further trials of therapies for these patients remains undiminished. However, there will be an increasing need for trials of anti-HIV agents in asymptomatic patients. Many of the infectious complications of HIV infection are reactivations of latent infections whose clinical manifestations are unmasked by disrupted immune function. Alongside specific anti-HIV therapy we will need to discover ways of identifying patients at risk of these reactivations and conduct trials of preventive interventions. There are already parallels to this approach in other immunocompromised patients, and physicians dealing with HIV should co-ordinate their experiences with those of physicians who have been dealing with immunocompromise for some time, most notably in the field of tissue transplantation. While we can expect further progress with the use of nucleoside analogues such as DDI, DDC and Zidovudine in various combinations, we can also look to the 1990s for progress in immunotherapy and hope that experience with this can be extrapolated towards a vaccine.

ASPECTS OF CLINICAL MANAGEMENT FOR PARTICULAR PATIENT GROUPS

Although the broad perception of HIV as a relentlessly progressive immunological disorder is appropriate for all patients, aspects of the infection may differ for particular patient groups.

Women

As already indicated, HIV-infected women face the additional problem of cervical disease. The natural history is not yet properly defined, but patients should be encouraged to undergo frequent screening. They also face the issue of pregnancy more directly than men. Some may wish to become pregnant. Some discover they are HIV-positive once pregnant (or vice versa) and may wish to continue or terminate the pregnancy. Both options should be available. Present investigations do not suggest that pregnancy adversely influences the course of HIV infection. Similarly there is little evidence that HIV infection adversely affects the outcome of pregnancy. Outside of the risk of HIV transmission by breast-feeding that has already been mentioned, it appears that 13 to 39 per cent of babies born to HIV-infected mothers will be HIV-infected. The influence of drugs, both self-administered and prescribed, on the foetus should also be considered. Women with children, especially small children, have the problem of child care during hospital attendance, admission and investigation. Whether or not the children are HIV-infected, it may be very important for mothers and children to be admitted together. This may be commonplace in countries of the developing world, but where services for HIV-infected patients have been developed predominantly for homosexual men, as in Europe and North America, such facilities may not exist.

Children

It has already been mentioned that the clinical manifestations of HIV infection in children differ in many respects from those in adults. This is, to a large extent, reflected in the CDC case definitions of AIDS (CDC, 1987a). However, a few extra points bear emphasis. HIV infection in children leads to a failing immune system on the background of a developing individual. Whereas a large percentage of infections arising in adult immunocompromised patients may be reactivations, those arising in children will tend to be primary infections. This may lead to differences in presentation. The course of childhood viral illnesses may be altered by immunocompromise and vaccination schedules need careful consideration. Zidovudine is now recognized as of significant benefit in paediatric AIDS (Yarchoan *et al.*, 1987) and most children with AIDS are also offered prophylaxis against PCP. In addition to these approaches to paediatric AIDS that have been extrapolated from experience with adults some reports have indicated benefit from repeated immunoglobulin infusions.

Intravenous drug users

Providing medical care for intravenous drug users has always been difficult. They are often irregular attenders at clinics and tend to present late with symptoms. In addition, the drug habit has often led to a deterioration in, or destruction of, their normal social support network of family, friends, employment and income. The question of breaking the law often arises and may prove particularly difficult with the prescription of opiates by the attending physician. The emphasis of registered prescribing for drug users with the Home Office has been to include these patients in drug-withdrawal programmes. This emphasis on withdrawal becomes less important for patients with what is a terminal disease. In many cases regular methadone prescription can provide a routine medical contact in what are often very chaotic lifestyles. In addition to these difficulties, there are particular clinical problems with intravenous drug users. The care of HIV-infected individuals often requires blood sampling for laboratory tests: these samples can be very difficult to obtain in patients who have used drugs for some time and have damaged the superficial veins usually used for phlebotomy. In some cases large neck or groin veins must be used and specific expertise is required to obtain the samples. Patients may then attempt to use these veins for drug injection, sometimes with disastrous results. Local skin and subcutaneous infections are common in drug users who continue to inject without using sterile conditions. These, and the other infections well characterized in drug users, such as bacterial infection of the heart valves, may be more frequent and more difficult to treat in those patients who are immunocompromised by HIV infection.

Haemophiliacs

As a striking contrast to intravenous drug users, haemophiliacs are predominantly regular hospital attenders who have had to develop close links with medical personnel in order to manage their bleeding problems. They are also familiar with injection techniques and blood sampling. The general course of HIV infection in these patients has been very similar to that seen in homosexual men: there are, however, some particular points to make. Many very young haemophiliacs have been infected and have then faced the difficulties of haemophilia and HIV infection through growth and development. Their risk of significant bleeding has meant that invasive diagnostic techniques, especially those involving biopsy such as trans-bronchial biopsy in the lungs, have been inappropriate. Empirical therapy may be more appropriate in some cases. This problem with bleeding is particularly emphasized by the condition of HIV-induced reduction in blood platelet numbers (thrombocytopenia). HIV-infected haemophiliacs with this problem face increased risks of bleeding not only as a result of their haemophilia, but also because of their low platelet counts.

Immigrants and refugees

In the UK, a significant number of men and women infected with HIV are immigrants. The majority of these come from sub-Saharan Africa and acquired the virus through heterosexual contact. Their perception of the infection has been determined by their experience in Africa, where large numbers, at least in urban centres, are known to be HIV-infected and many families have lost relatives with the diarrhoeal and wasting syndromes associated with AIDS ('Slim Disease'). Stigma in their own community frequently leads to secrecy about their condition with family and friends. In addition to language barriers, cultural differences may prove difficult to manage in the UK health system. For example, the status of African women depends to a large extent on bearing children. Asymptomatic HIV-infected women may face inordinate pressure within their own community to become pregnant. The extended family system operates in lieu of 'social security' in Africa and patients transplanted out of this system find the health system of the UK difficult to use and understand. African men are particularly unwilling to seek medical advice. The majority of these immigrant patients also face particular difficulties with employment and housing. As already indicated, tuberculosis may be a particular problem in these patients along with other latent infections with a high prevalence in developing countries.

CONCLUSION

The medical management of HIV-infected patients has moved from crisis management to monitoring and early intervention. This requires physicians to make an assessment of the state of immune function in each HIV-infected patient which, in turn, requires a combination of clinical skill and laboratory expertise. The more reliable this assessment is, the easier it is to tailor the main thrust of medical intervention to the patient's needs, be it towards active investigation and diagnosis or symptom control. In the 1990s physicians will be looking increasingly for ways of improving the tools available for assessing immune function and for agents other than nucleoside analogues that will be useful against HIV.

References

American Psychiatric Association. (1988) AIDS policy: confidentiality and disclosure. *American Journal of Psychiatry*, 145, 541–2.

Andolfi, M. (1980) Prescribing the family's own dysfunctional rules as therapeutic strategy. *Journal of Marital and Family Therapy*, 7, 255–64.

Andolfi, M., Angelo, C., Menghi, P. *et al.* (1983) *Behind the Family Mask: Therapeutic Change in Rigid Family Systems.* New York: Bruner Mazel.

Barbacci, M., Dalabeta, G., Repke, J., *et al.* (1990) Human immunodeficiency virus infection in women attending an inner-city prenatal clinic: ineffectedness of targeted screening. *Sexually Transmitted Diseases*, 17, 122–6.

Barre-Sinoussi, F., Cherman, J., Rey, F. *et al.* (1983) Isolation of a T-Lymphotropic retro-virus from a patient at risk for acquired immune deficiency syndrome (AIDS). *Science*, 220, 868–71.

Bateson, G. (1979) *Mind and Nature.* New York: Dutton.

Bayer, R., Levine, C. and Wolf, S. (1986) HIV antibody screening: an ethical framework for evaluating proposed programs. *Journal of the American Medical Association*, 256, 1768–74.

Beral, V., Peterman, T. A., Berkelman, R. L. and Jaffe, H. W. (1990) Kaposi's sarcoma among persons with AIDS: a sexually transmitted infection? *Lancet*, 335, 123–8.

Binder, R. (1987) AIDS antibody tests on inpatient psychiatric units. *American Journal of Psychiatry*, 144, 176–81.

Black, P. and Levy, E. (1988) HIV infection during pregnancy: psychosocial factors and medical implications. In R. Schinazi and A. Nahmias (Eds), *AIDS in Children, Adolescents and Heterosexual Adults.* New York: Elsevier.

Blanche, S., Rouzioux, C., Guihard, M. *et al.* (1989) A prospective study of infants born to women seropositive for human immuno-deficiency virus Type 1. *New England Journal of Medicine*, 320, 1643–8.

Bofill, M., Janossy, G., Lee, C. A., *et al.* (1992) Laboratory control values for CD4 and CD8 T lymphocytes – implications for HIV-1 diagnosis. *Clinical and Experimental Immunology*, 87, 1–10.

Bor, R. and Miller, R. (1990) *Internal Consultation in Health Care Settings.* London: Karnac Books.

Bor, R., Miller, R., Goldman, E. and Kernoff, P. (1989) The impact of AIDS/HIV on the family: themes emerging from family interviews. *Practice* 1, 42–8.

Bor, R., Miller, R. and Perry, L. (1988) Systemic counselling for patients with AIDS/HIV infections. *Family Systems Medicine*, 6, 21–39.

Bowen, S. and Michal-Johnson, P. (1988) The crisis of communicating in relationships: confronting the threat of AIDS. *AIDS and Public Policy Journal*, 4, 10–19.

Bozzette, S. A., Sattler, F. R., Chiu, J. *et al.* (1990) A controlled trial of early adjunctive treatment with corticosteroids for *Pneumocystis carinii* pneumonia in the acquired immuno-deficiency syndrome. California Collaborative Treatment Group. *New England Journal of Medicine*, 323, 1451–7.

Bradbeer, C. (1989) Women and HIV. *British Medical Journal*, 298, 342–3.

Branwhite, T. (1991) A question of change. *Counselling Psychology Review*, 6, 11–19.

British Medical Association. (1987) HIV antibody testing. *British Medical Journal*, 295, 911–13.

Buckman, R. (1984) Breaking bad news: why is it still so difficult? *British Medical Journal*, 288, 1597–99.

Burke, D. S., Brundage, J. F., Redfield, R. R. *et al.* (1988) Measurement of the false positive rate in a screening program for human immuno-deficiency virus infections. *New England Journal of Medicine*, 319, 961–4.

Campbell, D. and Draper, R. (1985) *Applications of Systemic Family Therapy: The Milan Approach.* London: Grune and Stratton.

Carballo, M. and Miller, D. (1989) HIV coun-selling: problems and opportunities in defining the agenda for the 1990s. *AIDS Care*, 1, 117–23.

Carter, B. and McGoldrick, M. (1989) *The Changing Family Life Cycle.* (2nd edn) Boston: Allyn and Bacon.

CDC (1986) Classification system for human T-lymphotropic virus type III/lymphadenopathy-associated virus infections. *Morbidity and Mortality Weekly Report*, **35**, 334–9.

CDC (1987a) Revision of the CDC surveillance case definition for acquired immunodeficiency syndrome. *Morbidity and Mortality Weekly Report*, **36**, 1S–15S.

CDC (1987b) Classification system for HIV in children less than 13 years of age. *Morbidity and Mortality Weekly Report*, **36**, 225–36.

CDC (1989) Guidelines for prophylaxis against *Pneumocystis carinii* pneumonia for persons infected with human immunodeficiency virus. *Morbidity and Mortality Weekly Report*, **38** Suppl 5, 1–9.

Cecchin, G. (1987) Hypothesizing, circularity, neutrality revisited: an invitation to curiosity. *Family Process*, **26**, 405–13.

Combrinck-Graham, L. (1987) Invitation to a kiss: diagnosing ecosystemically. *Psychotherapy*, **24**, 504–10.

Cooley, T. P., Kunches, L. M., Saunders, C. A. et al., (1990) Once-daily administration of 2',3'-dideoxyinosine (ddI) in patients with the acquired immunodeficiency syndrome or AIDS-related complex. Results of a Phase I trial. *New England Journal of Medicine*, **332**, 1340–5.

Courgnaud, V., Laure, F., Brossard, A. et al. (1991) Frequent and early *in utero* HIV-1 infection. *AIDS Research and Human Retroviruses*, 337–41.

Crowe, S., Stewart, K., Carlin, J. et al. (1990) Relationship between opportunistic infections (OI) and malignancy (OM) in HIV patients and CD4 lymphocyte number. *Sixth International Conference on AIDS*, San Francisco, SB526. (Abstract)

De Cock, K. M., Selick, R. M., Soro, B. et al. (1992) AIDS surveillance in Africa: a reappraisal of case definitions. *British Medical Journal*, **303**, 1185–8.

DHSS (1985) Information for doctors concerning the introduction of the HTLV 111 antibody test. *AIDS Booklet 2*, London: DHSS.

Dickens, B. (1988) Legal right and duties in the AIDS epidemic. *Science*, **239**, 580–6.

Ehrnst, A., Lindgren, S., Dictor, M. et al. (1991) HIV in pregnant women and their offspring: evidence for late transmission. *Lancet*, **338**, 203–7.

Elliott, M. W., Steven, M. H., Philips, G. D. et al. (1990) Non-invasive mechanical ventilation for acute respiratory failure. *British Medical Journal*, 358–60.

Elder, G. and Sever, J. (1988) AIDS and neurological disorders: an overview. *Annals of Neurology*, **23** (Suppl.), S4–S6, 187.

European Collaborative Study. (1991) Mother to child transmission of HIV infection. *Lancet*, **2**, 1039–42.

European Collaborative Study. (1991) Children born to women with HIV–1 infection: natural history and risk of transmission. *Lancet*, **337**, 253–60.

Eyster, M., Ballard, J., Gail, M. et al. (1989) Predictive markers for the acquired immunodeficiency syndrome (AIDS) in haemophiliacs: persistence of p24 antigen and low T4 cell count. *Annals of Internal Medicine*, **110**, 963–9.

Fahrner, R., Clement, M., Kline, A. et al. (1987) Helping young people face death: resuscitation status and outcome in first episode *Pneumocystis carinii* pneumonia. Abstract from the *3rd International Conference on AIDS*, Washington, DC.

Falloon, J., Kovacs, J., Hughes, W. et al. (1991) A preliminary evaluation of 566C80 for the treatment of *Pneumocystis* pneumonia in patients with the acquired immunodeficiency syndrome. *New England Journal of Medicine*, 1534–8.

Feigal, D. W., Katz, M. H., Greenspan, D. et al. (1991) The prevalence of oral lesions in HIV-infected homosexual and bisexual men – three San Francisco epidemiological cohorts. *AIDS*, **5**, 519–25.

Feinberg, P. (1990) Circular questions: establishing the relational context. *Family Systems Medicine*, **8**, 273–7.

Fischl, M. A., Richman, D. D., Grieco, M. H. et al. (1987) The efficacy of azidothymidine (AZT) in the treatment of patients with AIDS and AIDS-related complex. A double-blind, placebo-controlled trial. *New England Journal of Medicine*, **317**, 185–91.

Fischl, M. A., Parker, C. B., Pettinelli, C. et al. (1990a) A randomized controlled trial of a reduced daily dose of zidovudine in patients with the acquired immunodeficiency syndrome. The AIDS Clinical Trials Group. *New England Journal of Medicine*, **323**, 1009–14.

Fischl, M. A., Richman, D. D., Hansen, N. et al. (1990b) The safety and efficacy of zidovudine (AZT) in the treatment of subjects with mildly symptomatic human immunodeficiency virus Type 1 (HIV) infection. A double-bind, placebo-controlled trial. The AIDS Clinical

Trials Group. *Annals of Internal Medicine*, **112**, 727–37.

Fleuridas, C., Nelson, T., and Rosenthal, D. (1986) The evolution of circular questions: training family therapists. *Journal of Marital and Family Therapy*, **12**, 113–27.

Friedman, Y., Franklin, C., Freels, S. *et al.* (1991) Long-term survival of patients with AIDS, *Pneumocystis carinii* pneumonia and respiratory failure. *Journal of the American Medical Association*, **266**, 89–92.

Gagnon, S., Boota, A. M., Fischl, M. A. *et al.* (1990) Corticosteroids as adjunctive therapy for severe *Pneumocystis carinii* pneumonia in the acquired immunodeficiency syndrome. A double-bind, placebo-controlled trial. *New England Journal of Medicine*, **323**, 1444–50.

Gallo, D., Diggs, J. L., Shell, G. R. *et al.* (1986) Comparison of detection of antibody to the acquired immune deficiency syndrome virus by enzyme immunoassay, immunofluorescence, and Western blot methods. *Journal of Clinical Microbiology*, **23**, 1049–51.

Gillon, R. (1987) Testing for HIV without permission. *British Medical Journal*, **294**, 821–3.

Girardi, J., Keese, R. and Traver, L. (1988) Psychotherapist responsibility in notifying individuals at risk for exposure to HIV. *Journal of Sex Research*, **25**, 1–27.

Goolishian, H. and Anderson, H. (1987) Language systems and therapy: an evolving idea. *Psychotherapy*, **24**, 529–38.

Green, J. and Sherr, L. (1989) Dying, bereavement and loss. In J. Green and A. McCreaner (Eds), *Counselling in HIV and AIDS*. Oxford: Blackwell Scientific Publishers.

Harries, A. D. (1990) Tuberculosis and human immunodeficiency virus infection in developing countries. *Lancet*, **335**, 387–90.

Harrison, A. (1988). The emotional impact of a vascular birthmark. In J. Mulliken and A. Young (Eds), *Vascular Birthmarks*. London: W.B. Saunders.

Haseltine, W. A. (1989) Silent HIV infections. *New England Journal of Medicine*, **320**, 487–89.

Hingson, R., Strunen, L. and Berlin, B. (1990) Acquired immunodeficiency syndrome transmission: changes in knowledge and behaviour among teenagers. Massachusetts Statewide Surveys, 1986–1988. *Paediatrics*, **85**, 24–8.

Hino, S., Sugiyama, H., Doi, H. *et al.* (1987) Breaking the cycle of HTLV-1 transmission via carrier mothers' milk. *Lancet*, **2**, 158–9.

Hira, S., Kamanga, J., Bhat, G. *et al.* (1989) Perinatal transmission of HIV 1 in Zambia. *British Medical Journal*, **299**, 1250–2.

Hoffman, L. (1981) *Foundations of Family Therapy*. New York: Basic Books.

Holliman, R. E., Johnson, J. D., Gillespie, S. H. *et al.* (1991) New methods in the diagnosis and management of cerebral toxoplasmosis associated with the acquired immune deficiency syndrome. *Journal of Infection*, **23**, 281–5.

Hoy, A. (1985) Breaking bad news to patients. *British Journal of Hospital Medicine*, **8**, 96–9.

Jacobson, M. A., Bacchetti, P., Kolokathis, A. *et al.* (1991a) Surrogate markers for survival in patients with AIDS and AIDS-related complex treated with zidovudine. *British Medical Journal*, **302**, 73–8.

Jacobson, M. A., Mills, J., Rush, J., *et al.* (1991b) Morbidity and mortality of patients with AIDS and first-episode *Pneumocystis carinii* pneumonia unaffected by concomitant pulmonary cytomegalovirus infection. *American Review of Respiratory Disorders*, **144**, 6–9.

Jason, J. and Evatt, B. (1990) Pregnancies in human immune deficiency virus-infected sex partners of haemophilic men. *Archives of Diseases of Childhood*, **144**, 484–90.

Johnson, M. (1989) Human deficiency virus infection in women. *British Journal of Obstetrics and Gynaecology*, **96**, 11–14.

Karpel, M. (1980) Family secrets: 1. Conceptual and ethical issues in the relational context. 2. Ethical and practical considerations in therapeutic management. *Family Process*, **19**, 295–306.

Keeney, B. (1983) *Aesthetics of Change*. New York: Guildford Press.

Keeney, B. (1979) Ecosystemic epistemology: an alternative paradigm for diagnosis. *Family Process*, **18**, 117–29.

Kelly, G. (1969) Man's construction of his alternatives. In B. Maher (Ed.), *Clinical Psychology and Personality: The Selected Papers of George Kelly*. New York: John Wiley.

Kipke, M., Futterman, D. and Hein, K. (1990) AIDS during adolescence. *Medical Clinics of North America*, **74**, 1149–67.

Kramer, A., Fuchas, D., Milstein, S. *et al.* (1988) Immunological and immunogenetic markers that model the risk of AIDS. *Abstract 779 of IV International Conference on AIDS*, Stockholm.

Kubler-Ross, E. (1970) *On Death and Dying*.

London: Tavistock Publishers.

Lambert, J. S., Seidlin, M., Reichman, R. C. et al. (1990) 2',3'-dideoxyinosine (ddI) in patients with the acquired immunodeficiency syndrome or AIDS-related complex. A phase I trial. *New England Journal of Medicine*, **322**, 1333–40.

Larder, B. A., Darby, G. and Richman, D. D. (1989) HIV with reduced sensitivity to zidovudine (AZT) isolated during prolonged therapy. *Science*, **243**, 1731–4.

Laure, F., Courgnaud, V., Rouzioux, C. et al. (1988) Detection of HIV-1 DNA in infants and children by means of the polymerase chain reaction. *Lancet*, **2**, 538–41.

Lee, C., Miller, R. and Goldman, E. (1989) Treatment dilemmas for HIV infection haemophiliacs. *AIDS Care*, **1**, 153–8.

Lefere, J., Salmon, D. and Couvouce, A. (1988) Evolution towards AIDS in HIV-infected individuals, *Lancet*, **3**, 1220–1.

Leigh, T. R., Parsons, P., Hume, C. et al. (1989) Sputum induction for diagnosis of *Pneumocystis carinii* pneumonia. *Lancet*, **2**, 205–6.

Leoung, G. S., Feigal, D. W. J., Montgomery, A. B. et al. (1990) Aerosolized pentamidine for prophylaxis against *Pneumocystis carinii* pneumonia. The San Francisco community prophylaxis trial. *New England Journal of Medicine*, **323**, 769–75.

Loche, M. and Mach, B. (1988) Identification of HIV-infected seronegative individuals by a direct diagnostic test based on hybridization to amplified viral DNA. *Lancet*, **2**, 418–21.

Marcus, J., Butler, C., Hittelman, J. et al. (1988) A study of the natural history and onset of neurological findings in infants at risk for developing AIDS. *Neurology*, **38** (Suppl. 1), 164.

Marcus, R. (1988) Surveillance of health care workers exposed to blood from patients infected with the human immunodeficiency virus. *New England Journal of Medicine*, **319**, 1118–23.

Mason, J., Joyce, P., Spering, R. et al. (1991) Incorporating HIV education and counselling into routine prenatal care: a program model. *AIDS Education and Prevention*, **3**, 118–23.

Maturana, H., Coddou, F. and Mendez, C. (1988) The bringing forth of pathology. *Irish Journal of Psychology*, **9**, 144–72.

Mauksch, L. and Roesler, T. (1990) Expanding the context of the patient's explanatory model using circular questioning. *Family Systems Medicine*, **8**, 3–13.

McGoldrick, M. and Gerson, R. (1985) *Genograms in Family Assessment*. New York: W. W. Norton.

McGuire, P, and Faulkner, A. (1988) Communicate with cancer patients 2: handling uncertainty, collusion and denial. *British Medical Journal*, **297**, 972–4.

McLauchlan, C. (1990) Handling distressed relatives and breaking bad news. *British Medical Journal*, **301**, 1145–9.

Metersky, M. L. and Catanzaro, A. (1991) Diagnostic approach to *Pneumocystis carinii* pneumonia in the setting of prophylactic aerosolized pentamidine. *Chest*, **100**, 1345–9.

Millar, A. B., Patou, G., Miller, R. F. et al. (1990) Cytomegalovirus in the lungs of patients with AIDS. Respiratory pathogen or passenger? *American Review of Respiratory Disorders.*, **141**, 1474–7.

Miller, R. and Bor, R. (1988) *AIDS: A Guide to Clinical Counselling*. London: Science Press.

Moss, A. and Bacchetti, P. (1989) Natural history of HIV infection. *AIDS*, **3**, 55–61.

Minor, J. R. (1991) Foscarnet versus ganciclovir in the management of cytomegalovirus disease in patients with AIDS. *American Journal of Hospital Pharmacy*, **48**, 2478–9.

Mortimer, P. P. and Parry, J. V. (1992) Non-invasive virological diagnosis: are saliva and urine specimens adequate substitutes for blood? *Reviews in Medical Virology*, **1**, 73–8.

Moss, A. R. and Bacchetti, P. (1989) Natural history of HIV infection. *AIDS*, **3**, 55–61.

Nicoli, F., Chave, B., Peragut, J. C. et al. (1992) Efficacy of cytarabine in progressive multifocal leucoencephalopathy in AIDS. *Lancet*, **339**, 306.

Nordic Medical Research Council HIV Therapy Group (1992) Double-blind dose-response study of zidovudine in AIDS and advanced HIV infection. *British Medical Journal*, **304**, 13–17.

Novick, B. and Rubinstein, A. (1987) AIDS: the paediatric perspective. *AIDS*, **1**, 3–7.

O'Farrell, N. (1989) Transmission of HIV: genital ulceration, sexual behaviour, and circumcision. *Lancet*, **2**, 1157.

Palestine, A. G., Polis, M. A., Desmet, M. D. et al. (1991) A randomized, controlled trial of Foscarnet in the treatment of cytomegalovirus retinitis in patients with AIDS. *Annals of Internal Medicine*, **115**, 665–73.

Parry, A. (1984) Maturation in Milan: recent developments in systemic therapy. *Journal of Strategic and Systemic Therapies*, **3**, 35–42.

Penn, P. (1982) Circular questioning. *Family Process*, **24**, 299–310.

Penn, P. (1985) Feed forward: future questions, future maps. *Family Process*, **24**, 299–310.

Perakyla, A. and Bor, R. (1991) Interactional problems of addressing 'dreaded issues.' *AIDS Care*, **2**, 325–38.

Phair, J., Munoz, A., Detels, R. *et al.* (1990) The risk of *Pneumocystis carinii* pneumonia among men infected with human immunodefiency virus type 1. Multicenter AIDS Cohort Study Group [see comments]. *New England Journal of Medicine*, **322**, 161–5.

Phillips, A. N., Lee, C. A., Elford, J. *et al.* (1991) Serial CD4 lymphocyte counts and development of AIDS. *Lancet*, **337**, 389–92.

Potts, M. (1992) Conference Report: Sixth International Conference on AIDS in Africa. *Lancet*, **339**, 238.

Price, J., Desmond, S. and Kukulka, G. (1985) High school students' perceptions and misconceptions of AIDS. *Journal of School Health*, **55**, 107–9.

Ranki, A., Valle, S. L., Krohn, M. *et al.* (1987) Long latency precedes overt seroconversion in sexually transmitted human-immunodeficiency-virus infection. *Lancet*, **2**, 589–93.

Redfield, R. R., Wright, D. C. and Tramont, E. C. (1986) The Walter Reed staging classification for HTLV-III-LAV infection. *New England Journal of Medicine*, **314**, 131–2.

Resnick, L., Berger, J., Shapshak, P. *et al.* (1988) Early penetration of blood brain barrier by HIV. *Neurology*, **38**, 9–14.

Richards, T. (1986) Don't tell me on a Friday. *British Medical Journal*, **292**, 943.

Richman, D. D., Fischl, M. A., Grieco, M. H. *et al.* (1987) The toxicity of azidothymidine (AZT) in the treatment of patients with AIDS and AIDS-related complex. A double-blind, placebo-controlled trial. *New England Journal of Medicine*, **317**, 192–7.

Rogers, C. (1951) *Client-Centred Therapy.* Boston: Houghton Mifflin.

Rolland, J. (1984) Toward a psychosocial typology of chronic and life threatening illness. *Family Systems Medicine*, **2**, 245–62.

Rolland, J. (1987) Chronic illness and the life cycle: a conceptual framework. *Family Process*, **26**, 203–21.

Rolland, J. (1990) Anticipatory loss: a family systems developmental framework. *Family Process*, **29**, 229–44.

Ruskin, J. and LaRiviere, M. (1991) Low-dose co-trimoxazole for prevention of *Pneumocystis carinii* pneumonia in human immodeficiency virus disease. *Lancet*, **337**, 468–71.

Rutherford, N. O'Malley, P. Lifson, A. *et al.* (1990) Natural history of HIV infection in a cohort of homosexual and bisexual men: clinical and immunologic outcome 1977–1990. *Abstracts of VI International AIDS Conference, San Francisco.* Abstract No. Th 33.

Salt, H., Miller, R., Perry, L. *et al.* (1989) Paradoxical interventions in counselling for people with an intractable AIDS-worry. *AIDS Care*, **1**, 39–44.

Samuel, Q. (1989) Our patient's lifestyle is their business. *British Medical Journal*, **298**, 59.

Scott, G. Hutto, C., Makuch, R. *et al.* (1989) Survival in children with perinatally acquired human immunodeficiency virus Type 1 infection. *New England Journal of Medicine*, **321**, 1791–6.

Selvini-Palazzoli, M. (Ed.) (1986) *The Hidden Games of Organizations.* New York: Pantheon Books.

Selvini-Palazzoli, M., Boscolo, L., Cecchin, G. *et al.* (1977) Family rituals: a powerful tool in family therapy. *Family Process*, **4**, 445–53.

Selvini-Palazzoli, M., Boscolo, L., Cecchin, G. *et al.* (1980a) The problem of the referring person. *Journal of Marital and Family Therapy*, **6**, 3–9.

Selvini-Palazzoli, M., Boscolo, L., Cecchin, G. *et al.* (1980b) Hypothesizing, circularity, neutrality: three guidelines for the conductor of the session. *Family Process*, **19**, 3–12.

Sherr, L. (1991) *HIV and AIDS in Mothers and Babies: A Guide to Counselling.* Oxford: Blackwell Publications.

Sifris, D. and Sher, R. (1988) B2 microglobulin levels as a prognostic indicator of the development of AIDS, *Abstract 2516 of IV International Conference on AIDS.* Stockholm.

Simpson, D. M. and Wolfe, D. E. (1991) Neuromuscular complications of HIV infection and its treatment. *AIDS*, **5**, 917–26.

Speck, P. (1991) Breaking bad news. *Nursing Times*, **87**, 24–5.

Squire, S. B., Elford, J., Bor, R. *et al.* (1991) Open access clinic providing HIV-1 antibody results on day of testing: the first twelve months. *British Medical Journal*, 302, 1383–6.

Squire, S. and Johnson, M. (1990) Early diagnosis of HIV infection. *British Journal of Hospital Medicine*, 4th July.

Squire, S. B., Lipman, M. C. I., Bagdades, E. K. *et al.* (1992) Severe cytomegalovirus pneumonitis in HIV-infected patients with higher than average CD4 counts. *Thorax.* (in press).

Strunen, L. and Hingson, R. (1987) Acquired immunodeficiency syndrome and adolescents: knowledge, beliefs, attitudes and behaviour. *Paediatrics*, 79, 825–8.

Tomm, K. (1987a) Interventive interviewing. Part 1: Strategizing as a fourth guideline for the therapist. *Family Process*, 26, 3–13.

Tomm, K. (1987b) Interventive interviewing. Part 2: Reflexive questioning as a means to enable self-healing. *Family Process*, 26, 167–83.

Tomm, K. (1988) Interventive interviewing. Part 3: Intending to ask lineal, circular or reflexive questions? *Family Process*, 27, 1–15.

Ultmann, M., Diamond, G., Ruff, H. *et al.* (1987) Developmental abnormalities in children with acquired immunodeficiency syndrome (AIDS): a follow-up study. *International Journal of Neuroscience*, 32, 661–7.

Van Trommel, M. (1983) The intake procedure placed within a systemic context. *Journal of Strategic and Systemic Therapies*, 2, 74–86.

Volberding, P. A., Lagakos, S. W., Koch, M. A. *et al.* (1990) Zidovudine in asymptomatic human immunodeficiency virus infection. A controlled trial in persons with fewer than 500 CD4-positive cells per cubic milimetre. The AIDS Clinical Trials Group of the National Institute of Allergy and Infectious Diseases. *New England Journal of Medicine*, 322, 941–9.

Walker, G. (1991) *In the Midst of Winter.* New York: W. W. Norton.

Watzlawick, P., Beaven, J. and Jackson, D. (1967) *Pragmatics of Human Communication.* New York: W. W. Norton.

Watzlawick, P., Weakland, J. and Fisch, R. (1974) *Change: Principles of Problem Formation and Problem Resolution.* New York: W. W. Norton.

Webster, A., Lee, C., Cook, D. *et al.* (1988) Cytomegalovirus infection and progression towards AIDS in haemophiliacs with human immunodeficiency virus infection, *Lancet*, ii, 63–6.

Welch-Cline, R. (1988) Communication and death and dying: implications for coping with AIDS. *AIDS and Public Policy Journal*, 4, 40–50.

WHO (1990) *Guidelines for counselling people about HIV.* Geneva: World Health Organization.

Yarchoan, R., Berg, G., Brouwers, P. *et al.* (1987) Response of human-immunodeficiency-virus-associated neurological disease in 3'-azido-3'-deoxythymidine. *Lancet*, 1, 132–5.

Young, D. and Beier, E. (1982) Being asocial in social places: giving the client a new experience. In J. Anchin and D. Kiesler (Eds), *Handbook of Interpersonal Psychotherapy.* New York: Pergamon.

Index